Advance Praise
THE REDUCETARIAN SOLUTION

"This book offers us a path toward a more ecological, sustainable, humane, and compassionate world while improving our own health and well-being."
—Deepak Chopra, author of *Quantum Healing*

"Brian is a true visionary—a courageous leader of wellness and compassion. His practical advice and delicious yet simple recipes in *The Reducetarian Solution* will inspire you to transform the way you live, love, and eat."
—Kris Carr, wellness activist and *New York Times* best-selling author of *Crazy Sexy Diet*

"Reducetarianism: 2 → 1 burgers saves as many cows as 1 → 0."
—Steven Pinker, author of *The Better Angels of Our Nature: Why Violence Has Declined*

"*The Reducetarian Solution* is a bold new blueprint for a healthier and more compassionate food system, one conscious consumers and businesses are increasingly adopting."
—John Mackey, co-founder and co-CEO of Whole Foods Market

"Full vegetarianism is a noble ideal, but many are intimidated by an illogical fear that it has to be a single major, all-or-nothing leap. Reducetarianism is a good, humane, environment-friendly, step-by-step approach to an idea whose time will finally come."
—Richard Dawkins, author of *The God Delusion*, *An Appetite for Wonder*, and *Brief Candle in the Dark*

"Moderation in everything means being a reducetarian in practice. By eating less meat, you'll be doing your body, your planet, and your kids' future a favor. And you'll be proving once again that small steps can take us long distances."
—Daniel H. Pink, author of *Drive* and *A Whole New Mind*

"*The Reducetarian Solution* reveals a practical way to address the moral case for animal rights, sparing farm animals from suffering, and preserving the environment from destruction."
—Noam Chomsky, author of *Profit Over People: Neoliberalism & Global Order*

"The Reducetarian movement has the power to make us all—'all' meaning ourselves, our children, and millions and millions of suffering animals—happier and healthier."
—Susan Cain, *New York Times* best-selling author of *Quiet: The Power of Introverts in a World That Can't Stop Talking*

"A balanced mood, energized body, and sharp brain are just a few of the many benefits of being a reducetarian."
—Sonja Lyubomirsky, author of *The How of Happiness*

"Reducetarianism reminds us that progress is achieved incrementally. The very idea empowers everyone to participate in saving the world."
—Andrew Solomon, author of *Far from the Tree: Parents, Children, and the Search for Identity*

"*The Reducetarian Solution* shines a spotlight on proven and time-tested tips that will help you master a delicious, healthy, and compassionate lifestyle. If you are interested in unleashing your own creativity in the kitchen, you'll want to read this book!"
—Scott Barry Kaufman, author of *Wired to Create: Unraveling the Mysteries of the Creative Mind*

"This life-changing book is all about the power you have, right now, to gain more physical, mental, social, and spiritual strength—by reducing one thing, one simple thing. If you're looking for a way to live life more fully, following the advice in this book is probably the single smartest strategy you could adopt."
—Jane McGonigal, PhD, author of *SuperBetter* and *Reality Is Broken*

"Here is a simple, smart, world-changing practice that does not require me to entirely give up pork tacos. Kudos, Brian Kateman!"
—Mary Roach, author of *Gulp: Adventures on the Alimentary Canal*

"It's easy to operate on autopilot, making choices out of habit. Thank you Reducetarian movement for reminding us to eat with a little more deliberation."
—David Eagleman, neuroscientist and author of *The Brain*

"Many of us are troubled by the fact that, given current farming practices, our dietary choices impose continuous suffering on billions of non-human animals. However, there is an easy way to be less complicit in this misery: become a 'reducetarian' and eat less meat."
—Sam Harris, author of *Waking Up: A Guide to Spirituality without Religion*

"The one thing that everybody agrees on is that vegetables are a boon to health. This book offers great ideas for how to eat more plants, feel great, and improve your health."
—Tess Masters, author of *The Blender Girl*

"There are some ideas that make such obvious sense that one wonders why they haven't become universally adopted by now. Reducetarianism is one of them."

—Lawrence Krauss, author of *The Physics of Star Trek* and *A Universe from Nothing*

"*The Reducetarian Solution* is a game changer. It holds the key to a satisfying life and better world."

—Barry Schwartz, author of *The Paradox of Choice*

"Trying to be perfect can be paralyzing. But we have a natural capacity for goodness, and the insight behind the Reducetarian movement is that being just a little bit better—or even less terrible—can do wonders in lessening the suffering of helpless creatures."

—Paul Bloom, author of *Just Babies: The Origins of Good and Evil*

"*The Reducetarian Solution* blows the lid off of everything you thought you knew about meat."

—Martha Rosenberg, author of *Born with a Junk Food Deficiency: How Flaks, Quacks, and Hacks Pimp the Public Health*

"*The Reducetarian Solution* is a fresh and fascinating peek into how we change history through the surprising power of small acts that unite people in movements for social change."

—Dacher Keltner, author of *Born to Be Good: The Science of a Meaningful Life*

"Thanks to *The Reducetarian Solution*, it is now easier than ever to eat less meat and transform your life!"

—Chloe Coscarelli, author of *Chloe's Vegan Italian Kitchen*

"*The Reducetarian Solution* reminds us that there's a lot of deliciousness to be found outside the animal kingdom. If we can each eat just a little less meat than we do now, we can contribute to a tangible, positive change."

—Dan Pashman, host of *The Sporkful* food podcast and Cooking Channel's *You're Eating It Wrong*

"People will aggressively defend their choice of food because nothing speaks more strongly to people's identity. The power of this book and the reduction principle is that it recognizes this and reinforces the positive social values of food by challenging the waste of thoughtless, meaningless overconsumption."

—George Marshall, founder of Climate Outreach Information Network and author of *Don't Even Think About It: Why Our Brains Are Wired to Ignore Climate Change*

"What we eat has a big impact on the planet. We all need to do our bit, and this book shows you how."
> —Mark Miodownik, author of *Stuff Matters: Exploring the Marvelous Materials That Shape Our Man-Made World*

"Want to live a longer, healthier, and happier life? This book is for you."
> —Michael Greger, co-author of *How Not to Die: Discover the Foods Scientifically Proven to Prevent and Reverse Diseases*

"*The Reducetarian Solution* serves as an important reminder that we are all part of one planet and must work together to achieve a sustainable, more equitable society."
> —Paul Ehrlich, author of *The Population Bomb*

"A witty, informative, and engaging book, *The Reducetarian Solution* is overflowing with simple suggestions to transform the way we live and manage ourselves."
> —Gernot Wagner, coauthor of *Climate Shock: The Economic Consequences of a Hotter Planet*

"Incremental change, enacted on a broad enough scale, beats radical utopianism every time. Here is a great big book on how to do things smaller."
> —Douglas Rushkoff, author of *Throwing Rocks at the Google Bus* and *Present Shock*

"*The Reducetarian Solution* is non-dogmatic; it sets admirable goals for the billions of humans who aren't willing to stop eating meat entirely."
> —Adam Atler, author of *Drunk Tank Pink*

"I have seen the future and it is filled with reducetarians. Reducing the amount of meat we eat will selfishly benefit us as it selflessly benefits the planet."
> —Brian Wansink, author of *Slim by Design: Mindless Eating Solutions for Everyday Life*

"With great wisdom and humor, Brian Kateman unmasks a subtle but powerful notion: a small change among many is often more transformative than a large change among a few."
> —Jonah Berger, best-selling author of *Invisible Influence* and *Contagious: Why Things Catch On*

"*The Reducetarian Solution* has transformative potential for our planet because it puts change within reach of everyone, not just the most zealous or the most committed."
> —Christian Rudder, cofounder of OkCupid and author of *Dataclysm: Love, Sex, Race, and Identity—What Our Online Lives Tell Us about Our Offline Selves*

THE
REDUCETARIAN
SOLUTION

THE
REDUCETARIAN
SOLUTION

How the Surprisingly Simple Act of
Reducing the Amount of Meat in Your Diet
Can Transform Your Health and the Planet

Edited by Brian Kateman

Foreword by Mark Bittman

Recipes by Pat Crocker

A TarcherPerigee Book

tarcherperigee

An imprint of Penguin Random House LLC
375 Hudson Street
New York, New York 10014

Most TarcherPerigee books are available at special quantity discounts for bulk purchase for sales promotions, premiums, fund-raising, and educational needs. Special books or book excerpts also can be created to fit specific needs. For details, write: SpecialMarkets@penguinrandomhouse.com.

LIBRARY OF CONGRESS CATALOGING-IN-PUBLICATION DATA
Names: Kateman, Brian, editor.
Title: The reducetarian solution : how the surprisingly simple act of
 reducing the amount of meat in your diet can transform your health and the
 planet / edited by Brian Kateman ; foreword by Mark Bittman ; recipes by
 Pat Crocker.
Description: New York, New York : TarcherPerigee, [2017] | Includes index.
Identifiers: LCCN 2016050531 | ISBN 9780143129714 (paperback)
Subjects: LCSH: Nutrition—Popular works. | Food habits—Popular works. |
 Meat—Health aspects. | Vegetarianism—Health aspects. | Self-care,
 Health—Popular works. | BISAC: HEALTH & FITNESS / Diets. | HEALTH &
 FITNESS / Healthy Living. | COOKING / Essays.
Classification: LCC RA784 .R435 2017 | DDC 613.2—dc23
LC record available at https://lccn.loc.gov/2016050531

Printed in the United States of America

10 9 8 7 6 5 4 3 2 1

Book design by Sabrina Bowers

CONTENTS

MIND

BODY

PLANET

FOREWORD

■ Mark Bittman

It's difficult to believe there are many people remaining in the United States who do not yet understand this message: Eat less meat, and both you and the planet will benefit. There are few other changes you can make in your life that will allow you to be both selfish and altruistic at the same time. And yet, becoming a reducetarian does just that, by helping you reduce both your chances of chronic disease and also your carbon footprint and the other damaging environmental consequences of industrial animal production.

It's true that the word itself—*reducetarian*—is a relatively new one. Whether it replaces or complements flexitarian (which is less specific), less-meatarian (roughly equivalent), vegetarian (somewhat stricter), or vegan (much stricter) remains to be seen. But ultimately, it's not the label or the logistic details that matter here. Whether you "do" Meatless Monday or Vegan before 6 (invented by me!) or some other strategy designed to cut down on your meat consumption is equally immaterial. What matters is that people begin to act on a reality that's become increasingly clear and consistently proven by fact.

What follows is a series of fine essays that make this point in many different ways, written by an all-star cast. Among the writers are friends, colleagues, and people I've admired from afar. Today we move increasingly toward a precipice—it is a far different place from where were stood just a few years ago. In widening circles, eating less meat is becoming more and more common. And as I've already said, the benefits of reducetarianism are no longer in dispute.

Still, Big Food is a powerful lobby and will go to almost any lengths to protect its position; it's telling that almost no politicians are actually willing to come out and say "excessive meat consumption is bad." And so, despite the fact that so many people know that the current state of food is bad for us, it retains many loyal defenders. (In this

way, it's a lot like American football.) This is one of the things that
make *The Reducetarian Solution* so valuable: It counters, from many
angles, the notion that the status quo is acceptable. We have to make
a change—and fast. This book, with its mission to help make that
change, will be worth reading more than once.

INTRODUCTION

■ Brian Kateman

On a hot summer afternoon in Manhattan, my friend Tyler Alterman and I met for our weekly lunch. Tyler often writes at the Hungarian Pastry Shop, a cozy, dimly lit café near my office at Columbia University, so we decided to meet on the steps of the Cathedral of Saint John the Divine just across the street. He noticed I had brought a chicken salad and was surprised by my choice. "Aren't you a vegetarian?" he asked somewhat sheepishly. I explained to him that I wasn't a vegetarian but was eating more plant-based meals and was gradually decreasing my meat consumption to improve my health. Tyler shared that he also had been cutting down on meat, for animal welfare reasons, but had difficulty explaining his efforts to others.

From conversations that we've had with friends and colleagues, we realized we weren't alone. There was a growing community of individuals who knew that large-scale meat production and consumption was responsible for a significant amount of global greenhouse gas emissions, for poor health, and for the suffering of animals. And yet they weren't able or willing to completely eliminate meat from their diet. Some enjoyed the taste of meat; others didn't want to make a drastic lifestyle change. So they took the advice of Michael Pollan: "Eat food. Not too much. Mostly plants." They relied on useful strategies like Meatless Monday and Vegan before 6 to eat less meat for the benefit of themselves and for their environment.

They knew eating less meat made a meaningful difference, but they still struggled to describe their eating choices, particularly to vegans and vegetarians, the modern day pioneers of abstaining from meat and animal products.

These individuals were not vegetarians or vegans or even on any particular diet. And while they knew of terms like *semi-vegetarian* and *mostly vegetarian*, they struggled to adopt them as identities because they were exclusive to people who primarily followed a plant-based diet and seemed morally weak and behaviorally inconsistent. It is true that these identities guide incredibly positive steps toward a more sustainable planet, but for many, they invoke negative associations, feelings of division, and moral incompatibility.

Tyler and I realized there was a need for a term for people like us, people who take action to reduce their meat consumption, no matter the degree or motivation. After many brainstorming sessions, in the summer of 2014 we finally came up with the term *reducetarian* to describe a person who is simply committed to eating less meat. This is how the Reducetarian movement was born.

Reducetarianism is an identity, a community, and a movement. It is composed of individuals who are committed to eating less meat—red meat, poultry, and seafood. It challenges the notion that the only way to reap the benefits of reducing meat consumption is to eliminate meat from our lives entirely and recognizes that people are at different stages of willingness and commitment to eating less meat.

Reducetarianism is inclusive in that vegans and vegetarians are also reducetarians because they too have reduced their meat consumption. It unites the growing community of individuals who are committed to eating less meat and ends what can sometimes feel like a battle among vegans, vegetarians, and all those reducing their consumption of meat. This new perspective provides everyone with a platform—not just vegans and vegetarians—to make small choices to eat less meat in their own lives and collectively to make huge differences in the world.

With less meat and more fruits, vegetables, whole grains, and plant-based proteins such as beans and lentils, reducetarians live longer, healthier, and happier lives. Dr. Michael Orlich and colleagues of Loma Linda University found that among 73,308 Seventh-Day Adventist men and women, compared to typical omnivores, those who ate less meat had up to a 15 percent lower risk of death.[1] In fact, eating less meat and more whole, plant-based foods is one of the lifestyle habits that unites the people living to 100 and beyond in hot spots of longevity—regions called Blue Zones. Reducetarians enjoy these benefits by setting manageable and therefore actionable goals to gradually eat less meat. For example, they may forego eating meat for lunch if they will have it for dinner, skip eating meat on Mondays, or eat it only on the weekends.

Reducetarians know that eating less meat is good not only for themselves but also for the well-being of animals and the planet. Did you know that the average American eats approximately 2,000 land animals in his or her lifetime, leading to the suffering of over 9 billion factory-farmed animals every year in the United States alone?[2] The number of sea animals killed is so high that it's difficult to estimate. It's pretty simple: The less meat we eat, the more animals we save. And along the way, reducetarians mitigate water scarcity and climate change issues. Dr. Arjen Y. Hoekstra of the University of Twente in the Netherlands found that diets consisting of less meat could reduce food-related water footprints by up to 36 percent.[3] In a separate study, Dr. David Tilman and Mr. Michael Clark of the University of Minnesota calculated that eating more plant-based proteins could reduce greenhouse gas emissions by up to 55 percent.[4] There's no doubt about it—eating less meat and being a reducetarian is healthy, easy, and good.

This book is a compilation of perspectives from thought leaders across many disciplines on the concept of reducetarianism. The essays are categorized into three sections, (1) mind, (2) body, and (3) planet, as our food choices affect each in profound and distinct ways. The purpose of the book is to provide information and guidance on eating less meat. Along the way, you'll learn about the environmental, health, and animal welfare benefits of eating less meat; emerging trends in cutting-edge meat alternatives; how corporations and the economy shape meat consumption patterns; scientific and philosophical perspectives on meat, such as myths concerning meat consumption and human evolution; the relationship between meat and our far-distant galaxies; and more. Throughout, you will encounter strategies for eating less meat. And finally, you will discover easy vegan, vegetarian, and reduced-meat recipes to put reducetarianism into practice in your own life.

This array of perspectives on reducetarianism from influential thinkers around the world paired with simple and fun recipes from renowned chef Pat Crocker will provide you with useful tools and resources to eat less meat and encourage others to do the same.

Your journey to a healthier, more environmentally friendly, and compassionate lifestyle begins today—and once you've discovered how easy and impactful it can be, you'll want it to last forever.

MIND

The mind is everything. What you think you become.
—BUDDHA

THE BIZARRE FORCES THAT DRIVE PEOPLE TO EAT TOO MUCH MEAT

■ David Robinson Simon

Author of *Meatonomics: How the Rigged Economics of Meat and Dairy Make You Consume Too Much—and How to Eat Better, Live Longer, and Spend Smarter*

Americans consume almost 200 pounds of meat annually per person, more than almost any other people on the planet—and nearly twice what we ate 75 years ago.[1] We also have twice the incidence of diabetes and heart disease as the rest of the world and almost three times the incidence of cancer. There is little doubt that, as this book's many authors argue, we must reduce our meat consumption. Perhaps, like an engineer peering inside a motor to see how it works, we can explore the machinery of animal food production to learn *why* meat consumption levels are so high to begin with. If we can understand what makes Americans want to stuff a half pound of meat into our mouths every day, maybe we can find ways to cut those huge consumption levels.

As consumers, we like to think we make informed, well-founded decisions about what to buy. But when it comes to purchasing meat, new evidence shows consumers are routinely denied the ability to make such informed, rational decisions. Instead, government bureaucrats and industry players overwhelm consumers with a triple-whammy of price miscues, product misinformation, and aggressive manipulation. Like an invisible leash pulling us around by the neck, this set of influences literally changes our behavior and makes us buy more meat than otherwise. This essay looks at one of the most pernicious forces that drive people to consume animal foods in such huge quantities: artificially low prices.

THE DOUBLE $1 CHEESEBURGER

The price of a McDonald's double cheeseburger hasn't changed much in two and half decades—it was $1 in 1991, and it's just over $1 today. The prices of other consumer goods have increased substantially in that time. What keeps the price of meat so low?

The answer is *externalized costs*—a fancy term for a simple concept. Producers externalize their production costs when they impose them on society instead of bearing the costs themselves. Steve Wing, a University of North Carolina at Chapel Hill epidemiologist, expressed this phenomenon succinctly in a *New York Times* article published, serendipitously, the day I sat down to write this piece. "Pork is cheap and cheap to produce in large factories," said Wing, "because they don't pay for cleaning up the Des Moines water supply and they don't pay for the asthma neighbors get, they don't pay for polluting downstream water that used to be potable and they don't pay for the loss of property values." Couldn't have put it better myself.

The rise of factory farming over the past half century has, increasingly, given meat producers the means to externalize their production expenses and impose them on the rest of us. In my 2013 book *Meatonomics,* I add up these costs and find they total more than $414 billion. To put this huge number in perspective, it's about one quarter of Canada's gross domestic product or half of what the United States spends on Social Security each year.

Here's the rub: By massively externalizing their costs in this fashion, meat producers have been able to aggressively lower their products' prices. Thus, on an inflation-adjusted basis, the retail prices of various kinds of meat have fallen dramatically in the past half century. Since 1935, steak prices are down 20 percent, ham is down 48 percent, and chicken is down a whopping 74 percent.

It's hard to overstate the importance of a good's price when it comes to a consumer's decision to buy it or leave it. The most basic principle of economics, the *law of demand*, says that when a good's price is low, we'll likely buy more of it than if the price were higher. Pretty simple. But when it comes to meat prices, the result is shocking: Retail prices, pushed down to artificially low levels by producers' externalizing most of their production costs, cause Americans to eat much more meat than we would if prices rose to their true levels.

How do we know that low prices are driving high consumption? Because hundreds of studies have shown that consumption of animal foods is closely linked to price. On average, for every 10 percent drop in meat and dairy prices, consumption rises by about 6.5 percent. Conversely, if prices rise by 10 percent, consumption falls by about 6.5 percent. There are lots of reasons people buy meat: beliefs, preferences, disposable income, force of habit, and other factors. But the data on price and consumption show that retail prices play an enormous role. As animal science professor Marta Rivera-Ferre notes, "consumer demand [for meat] is not linked with the actual biological needs of the human organism *but with prices.*"[2]

REPAIRING THE DAMAGE

Now that we know why the market for animal foods is broken, we can also posit one easy way to fix it: Let meat prices rise to their true levels. For every dollar of animal foods sold at retail, another $1.70 is imposed on consumers and taxpayers in the form of externalized costs. This means that a $5 Big Mac really *costs* society $13. A $15 slab of ribs really *costs* $40. If the retail prices of these goods reflected their true societal cost, meat consumption would drop faster than you can say "tofu."

There are lots of ways to add externalized costs back into the retail price of meat. We might eliminate government subsidies, impose a tax on meat, or use other legislative or regulatory measures to force producers to bear their fair share of costs. In fact, any activity that raises the price of meat will help shift Americans' protein consumption to plant-based alternatives and would be a welcome step in the right direction. Most consumers *want* to act rationally. Let's make that possible by giving ourselves the proper price cues to do so.

THE ELEMENT OF SURPRISE

▊ Tania Luna

Co-author of *Surprise: Embrace the Unpredictable and Engineer the Unexpected*

It would be nice to be able to simply wake up one day and decide: "I'm going to eat less meat." But as my fellow humans know, things rarely work out that easily. Scientists suspect that one of the reasons we have a tough time changing our habits, even when we know they're bad for us, is that willpower—our internal voice of reason—is not unlimited. Just like any other resource, it can become depleted.

In an experiment by Roy Baumeister, participants waited in a room that smelled like freshly baked cookies. They were shown two types of foods: chocolates and radishes. Half of the participants were given chocolates and the other half got radishes. Next, researchers asked both groups to do a puzzle, and they timed how long it took participants to finish the task. The chocolate eaters kept trying for over eighteen minutes; the radish eaters quit after just eight.[1] Plenty of subsequent studies have since revealed the same concept: When we have to expend effort to regulate our impulses, we eventually run out of self-control.

But why does it take so much willpower to change how we eat? Part of the answer lies in habit. Habit is the enemy of change. Luckily for us, surprise is the enemy of habit. Most of our actions are patterns: We go home, sit on the couch, turn on the TV, think about food, get up to check the fridge, consider making a salad, feel tired and cranky—and end up grabbing the cold cuts.

It doesn't take a fortune-teller to predict the outcome of habitual actions because they contain no surprise. It's also an efficient way to live. Habits require less neural activity than new behaviors. But who wants efficiency when you can have excitement and fulfillment? (Okay, maybe you prefer efficiency, but it has its limits.) Surprise disrupts the pattern of habit, opening the door just a crack for new behaviors to slip in. Here are four tips for anyone attempting to disrupt their meat-eating habits.

1. SHAKE UP HOW YOU FEEL ABOUT FOOD.

Willpower is a fickle friend, but there is one exception: People who have strong beliefs can override even the coziest habits. How do you shake up your food feelings? Neuroscientist Wolfram Schultz found that surprise can intensify our emotions by about 400 percent,[2] creating just the kind of colorful memory that can act as your mouth's bouncer—keeping meat out when you don't want it in. So what might surprise you about food? Well, you can always Google "factory farming." A visit to a factory farm or slaughterhouse is another way to shock your system.

But there are also less emotionally scarring ways to surprise yourself. My husband, Brian, is from a part of Texas where *vegetarian* means "one of those people who's not from around here." Brian loves dogs, and intellectually, he knew that cows weren't much different, but it wasn't until he met a calf face to face for the first time recently that his perspective shifted. Rory the Calf had long, black lashes and a fuzzy nose; when she licked him, Brian fell in love. At the time we were traveling in Ireland, where burgers are served with nearly every meal, like napkins. After meeting Rory, however, Brian didn't want burgers. He's not a vegetarian, but now he doesn't eat beef. You could argue that he should be able to transfer his experience over to other animals. But that's just not how our brains always work. We need an emotional experience for that shift to happen.

2. MIX SURPRISE INTO YOUR SHOPPING.

Let's say you've shifted your thinking. That's step one. But how do you disrupt your old meat-eating habit even further? When willpower runs out, we've got to use our environment for help. The first place to mix in surprise is shopping. The more routine your trips to the supermarket are, the less room for change. So here are some very small ways to incorporate sparks of the unexpected into your list:

- Change the order of aisles you visit in the grocery store.
- Go to a different store.
- Always buy one non-meat food you've never tried.

- Visit farmers' markets and ask the vendors about their farms.
- Wear a reducetarian-inspired outfit while you shop. (Whatever that means to you!)

Yes, our brains love efficiency, but even more than that, they love novelty. New experiences release dopamine in our brains—the neurochemical that triggers excitement and pleasure. The more hits of dopamine you give your brain, the more motivated you'll be to keep up your surprising new approach to shopping.

3. "SURPRISIFY" YOUR KITCHEN.

Research shows that we make better food choices when we eat at home, but how can we get the most out of our home-cooked meals? As it turns out, a sprinkle of surprise works here too. Introduce novelty into your kitchen, and you'll be more likely to introduce novelty in your eating habits. The most effective changes are those that make eating meat a little harder and eating other foods a little easier (and more fun). Google used this technique when it realized employees were binging on M&Ms. First, managers placed the M&Ms in closed, opaque containers. Second, healthy snacks were placed in easy-to-reach areas. The result? In just seven weeks, Googlers consumed 3.1 million fewer calories (an average reduction of nine packages per employee).[3] Again, these aren't revolutionary switches, but they do cause us to pause. And within that pause, new behaviors have the opportunity to come alive. Here are a few other small surprise tweaks you can make this week:

- Use small skillets and plates for meat and large ones for everything else.
- Keep meat in a closed-off section of the fridge and fruits and veggies easily accessible.
- Purchase meat that isn't presliced.
- Buy beautiful (or funny) plates that you can use only when eating meat free.
- Make a relaxing or dance-inspiring playlist for healthy food prep. (Salad Songs?)
- Invite friends over to make and share meals together for the week.

- Create a theme for every month or even the year (for example, Moroccan March or The Year of the Homemade Salad Dressing).

4. TURN EATING AT RESTAURANTS INTO A GAME.

Last but not least, when eating out of the house, think about making the experience less about convenience and more about discovery. To really increase your dopamine levels, invite someone to join you. That way, you'll deepen your relationship as you collect surprising experiences together. A few tips for eating out:

- Ask the server to surprise you with a meat-free choice on the menu.
- Eat in a different way from the way you usually do (for example, with your hands, sitting on the floor).
- Share a plate of food and take turns tasting the same things at the same time.
- Have a blindfolded meal.

In short, take a look at your lifestyle. Where is there room for surprising, emotionally stirring experiences? Next, examine your eating habits. What's predictable? Make one small change per week and take note of which you enjoyed the most. Novelty boosts mood, and a positive mood increases willpower (making you even more capable of changing your habits). Plus surprise is fun, and who doesn't like fun? Now go on and surprise yourself.

A LITTLE LESS LONELY IN MY CORNER OF THE WORLD

Joanna Zelman

Executive editor at The Dodo

I was seven years old when I decided to reduce my meat consumption to help farm animals. It was 1993, a lonely time to embark on such an endeavor in my small town. The experience is different today. The rise of social media has pieced together those in many corners of the world who are passionate about animal welfare, the environment, and human health.

These online platforms are helping create a global community that can chip away at some of the loneliness many of us experienced: First graders clamoring for Big Mac toys surrounded me two decades ago. When I unwittingly ate a pepperoni-stuffed calzone, the entire lunchroom pointed and laughed. (Okay, it was possibly just the handful of first graders at my table who laughed. Or, maybe, it was even just one kid. But it felt as if the entire world were laughing at me.) I was fortunate to have an understanding family, but there were few resources and community support was scarce.

Now, we can Instagram veggie snacks, pin tasty dishes, and "like" a cauliflower casserole. We can pledge to join health challenges, blog our concerns for animals, and join meatless Twitter chats. Heck, we can even brag more. Tenth burger free Tuesday? Shout it from the rooftops! (Rooftops = Facebook status update.) And we can support each other's goals: comments, retweets, and likes are simple ways people are encouraging friends, family, and strangers to improve their health and the planet.

A decade ago, my (incredible!) mother would stock up on bags and bags of the only gelatin-free marshmallows we could find when we visited Washington, D.C. . . . six hours from home. These treats were so hard to come by that when I was roasting one marshmallow over a campfire and saw it melting into the flames, I lunged in and grabbed it with my bare hand. If only vegetarian marshmallows were an Amazon order away back then, I might have avoided wearing a burn bandage through the summer of 1999.

Access both to alternative products and to information have improved. We can find and share recipes online. Veggie-friendly restaurants are searchable by zip code. My friend on a budget wanted to reduce his meat consumption, so I sent him a Reddit thread of cheap vegan meals. We have easy access to advice from experts, like those at the Mayo Clinic encouraging meatless meals and the Centers for Disease and Control and Prevention's (CDC's) fruit and veggie recommendations. We can calculate our carbon footprint with the click of a button—and then realize that what we put in our mouth impacts the planet. When a family skips steak once a week, it's like taking their car off the road for almost three months.

Like all tools, those available in the digital age can be used for ill as easily as goodwill. The illegal wildlife trade and puppy mills have taken advantage of the Internet to the detriment of animals. Some viral videos even unknowingly promote the illegal pet trade, like of the slow loris. And cameras shut off when those "teacup pigs" suddenly start growing. Meanwhile, misinformation is rampant, and it's difficult to mine for the reputable animal care advice.

Demand for the newest, hottest, shiniest tech products to engage with our social media platforms are also demanding a lot from our planet's resources. Twice as many electronic products were sold in 2009 as in 1997, the EPA estimates—the sale of mobile devices increased nine times over.[1] Americans throw out millions of electronics every year, often without regard for proper e-waste disposal. This toxic waste threatens the health of millions of people around the world.

But it's far from all bad. Whistle-blower sites like WildLeaks, online resources to report animal cruelty, and access to tools protecting animals are helping out the good guys. It's easier to donate to reliable welfare groups. Undercover animal footage spreads rapidly (when it's not banned).

We've come a long way when it comes to getting big businesses to take notice.

I handwrote a letter to a major soup company in 1997, bemoaning their frequent use of animal stock. About two months later, I received coupons in the mail for beef soups. Now, thanks to online petitions, Twitterstorms, and calls to action, a company, politician, or influencer hears the concerns of thousands instantaneously. Digital advocacy and online campaigns can make it easier at times for voices to be heard.

For those who have never seen the faces before the meat, we now can. Stunning photos of cows helping their calves, videos that reveal a chicken's intelligence, Vines that capture the emotions of pigs—these can all now be found through sites like The Dodo, focused on helping the online community fall in love with animals.

Ultimately though, the lifestyle choices that affect our health, our animals, and our planet occur offline. Real-life interactions, be they of the human-human, human-animal, or human-nature variety, are invaluable.

Social media and online resources can help build communities, foster education, and spark empathy. But then let's look up from the screen, and share our experiences with those we can look straight in the eye and reach out to support.

CANNIBALISM IS NATURAL TOO

■ Richard Wrangham

Author of *Catching Fire: How Cooking Made Us Human*

Meat-eating is certainly natural, but that does not make it right.

It is almost forty years since I gave up red meat. During a three-year field study, I had watched chimpanzees rip the guts out of screaming, thrashing monkeys. The essential violence of carnivory was inescapable. I decided I would eat meat only if I was comfortable with imagining doing the killing myself. From feelings of empathy I determined not to eat mammals unless I was seriously hungry. The idea fit with my concerns about global ecology and personal health. It was an easy choice. Within a few years I cut back on birds and fish as well.

The decision to reduce meat consumption is no hardship if we live in affluent circumstances where meat is physiologically unnecessary and can even be bad for us. The prehistoric world was very different. Food was often scarce and meat gave important benefits. The same is true in some places today, such as where low-protein crops like cassava dominate the diet.

In the past, meat was important enough that its presence or absence at the evening meal would have affected everyone's happiness. Anthropologists have repeatedly recorded what happened when all of a camp's hunters failed. Without meat there was no feasting. Life lost its color and the mood was subdued.

Joy returned with the arrival of the next carcass. Around the fire there was singing and dancing and laughter. People regaled each other with stories of glorious hunts. They detailed the dramas of the kill and of the times when the prey dripped with fat. Once again the world became what hunter-gatherers believed it should always be, a place where people roasted animals every day.

All of us are descended from hunter-gatherers, and to judge from accounts of hunter-gatherer lives in every continent our ancestors would have had the same intense desire for meat and the same huge pleasure in eating it. Meat must have been a universal part of human happiness until very recently.

But evidence that some paleo diets were rich in meat is no excuse for eating it today, because we could make a similar argument about cannibalism.

Like other kinds of carnivory, cannibalism is a widespread natural behavior with adaptive benefits. Snails that eat their smaller siblings grow enormously faster than others. Insects thrive from eating eggs laid by their mothers. Some fish survive periods of food scarcity by eating their own young.

Adaptive cannibalism is practiced by many mammals. Primates such as our two closest relatives, chimpanzees and bonobos, readily eat their own. Mothers occasionally eat their infants, and adults of both sexes compete to eat unrelated youngsters that have been hunted and killed. Often not a scrap is left.

Humans seem to have followed the animal trend.[1] According to anthropologist Tim White, butchery of human bones indicates a deep history of frequent cannibalism. About 800,000 years ago in Atapuerca, northern Spain, crania and long bones of *Homo antecessor* were smashed and cut with stone tools as if to take brains, meat, and limb marrow. Around 100,000 years ago, French and Croatian Neanderthals cooked each other. A few hundred years ago in pre-Columbian Colorado, thousands of bone fragments show that people routinely used pots to cook and eat human flesh. Muscle protein in fossil feces provides the capstone evidence that butchering and cooking was accompanied by the eating of human meat.

In recent times cannibalism was found in the Americas, Africa, and New Guinea. These areas were invaded so late by European and Asian farmers that anthropologists were able to document the ancient habits. The practice held various kinds of symbolic value. Central American Aztecs sacrificed their enemies or made victims of religiously significant figures. The Fore of Papua New Guinea ate the brains of those who had died naturally.

The Fore case is particularly intriguing because it raises the possibility that our species has been so cannibalistic that we have adapted biologically to it. Many Fore cannibals acquired a disease called kuru, caused by a prion that passed from the eaten brain to the consumer. But some Fore cannibals were protected from kuru by a genetic adaptation of the *PRNP* gene, which gave resistance to prion diseases. The same genetic adaptation is widespread in much of the world. Conceivably our cannibalistic past has been so extensive that the entire human species has adapted to it.

Even today survival cannibalism can be acceptable. After a sperm whale sank the whaling ship *Essex* in 1820 the captain, George Pollard, drifted in a small boat in the Pacific with five other men. The first to die was eaten. Later, by agreement, the sailors drew lots to decide the next victim. The unlucky one was shot and cannibalized. In the end two survived and returned to Nantucket. According to Nathaniel Philbrick, the Quaker community there was intolerant of gambling, let alone homicide, but they accepted the logic of survival cannibalism even in the rare case when it involved taking a life. Pollard was awarded captaincy of another ship.

Cannibalism is a natural and adaptive behavior practiced by

many species, and it has a long history of being important in our own lineage. But we have come to regard it as immoral, so in most circumstances we are no longer cannibals.

Meat eating is likewise a widespread natural behavior that played a significant role in our evolutionary history. But as with cannibalism, that does not justify our being meat eaters.

Of course many people nowadays see a moral distinction between cannibalism and eating nonhuman mammals. But the difference is clearly subject to change. It was absent or greatly reduced in the past (when eating both our own and other species was considered to be legitimate), and I suspect it will be absent or greatly reduced in the future (when eating both our own and other species will be considered to be illegitimate).

For the moment, however, we are in an intermediate phase in which cannibalism and the eating of animal meat are often given a contrasting moral status.

For myself, I feel about eating mammals, parrots, and some other cognitively sophisticated species much as I do about human meat. Both kinds of food are natural and were probably relished by our ancestors. But in a world of nutritional plenty I do not need to eat either of them, and I prefer not to do so. I do not want to lower myself to the moral level of a monkey-eating chimpanzee or a cannibal ancestor. I believe that Katharine Hepburn's character had the right idea when she reprimanded the unsophisticated Charlie Allnut, played by Humphrey Bogart, in *The African Queen*: "Nature, Mr. Allnut, is what we were put on Earth to rise above."

ON WHERE AND HOW TO DRAW THE LINE

■ Dale Peterson

Author of *The Moral Lives of Animals*

Absolute rules are sometimes useful but often troublesome, and they can have the opposite effect of what they were intended to do. God's absolute prohibition against eating a piece of fruit in the Garden of Eden is what, so Christian preachers tell us, destroyed our original place in paradise. But who was really at fault there? Adam and Eve for succumbing to the temptation of an apparently special and probably delicious fruit? The evil serpent for sneakily stimulating that temptation? Or God, for establishing an absolute rule that was guaranteed to lead to temptation, followed by failure? Humans are perfectly imperfect—God should have known this, presumably, as he created us.

God was an Absolutarian. Adam and Eve, in all their imperfection, became Lapsarians. In doing so, they left the rest of humanity eternally in the lurch. One might call us the post-Lapsarians. There must be a better way.

I have called myself a vegetarian for many years now, inspired in part by the example of my friend Jane Goodall. Jane now and then scolds me for eating fish—in her opinion, this makes me something other than a vegetarian. I prefer to think of it as yet another example of the limits of absolutism. The fact is that I, like a lot of people, am not an Absolute Vegetarian. I am not ready to draw an absolute line, or at least not the sort of line that some people seem to expect.

But it would be a mistake, I think, to view this lack of absolutism as a failure. The human condition, as previously discussed, is anchored in the idea of fallibility. What's more important, then, is our ability to understand and justify our (often imperfect) actions. To know, in other words, where to draw the line.

For example, I draw the line at cannibalism. I don't know how to justify that decision logically. I simply draw the line at cannibalism based on the illogical but deeply felt sense that cannibalism is morally abhorrent. Indeed, the way I decide what meat I eat is tied closely to my views on evolutionary relationships. Similarly, because the evolutionary and genetic distinction between humans and the other great apes is really quite minor, I also would never eat great ape meat, since doing so would be far too close to cannibalism. Come to think of it, that is also why I would never eat any kind of primate meat, whether from monkeys, lemurs, beautiful golden lion tamarins, gorgeous Mentawai Island gibbons, and so on.

I am very cognizant of my identity as a mammal, something that also influences my decision making. I speak to dogs and expect them to understand—if not my words, then the feeling behind them. I'm not as close to cats, but my daughter and my sister-in-law are quite fond of them, an emotional connection I respect. Ultimately, I feel a strong basic kinship with dogs, cats, lions, giraffes, elephants, bumblebee bats, blue whales, and indeed all of the thousands of living species that belong to the magnificent mammalian class. I am a mammal and will not eat the meat of my fellow mammals. Mammals are not only my kin; they are my intelligent and potentially conscious kin. Here, again, is where I draw the line.

Thinking outside the mammalian box, my loyalties become increasingly idiosyncratic. I avoid eating birds because birds are wonderful and should be left alone. And also because of Irene Pepperberg, who seriously converses with parrots—although I will confess (throw stones if you must) that I eat white bird meat once a year at Thanksgiving.

Based on the kinship and consciousness concept, I could conceivably consume insects of any kind, and I also sometimes eat fish, though never lobsters and absolutely never octopus. The exceptions for lobsters and octopus come from general sympathy, intuition, and taste (lobsters are boiled alive and who would eat an octopus anyway?). Justifying this exception further, neuroscientist David Edelman has convinced me of the intelligence of octopuses, as has the author Sy Montgomery, who recently wrote a book about the "soul" of an octopus. Sy, it should be noted, has introduced me to a couple of very nice octopuses with real personalities at the New England Aquarium in Boston. And thus they remain on the safe side of my line.

TRICKED!

■ Seth Godin

Author of eighteen international best sellers including
All Marketers Are Liars: The Underground Classic That Ex-
plains How Marketing Really Works—and Why Authenticity
Is the Best Marketing of All

Consumers are getting smarter and more cynical, daily. We are better than ever at seeing through the corporate haze, and we don't
like being tricked, even though we still get fooled all the time.

The worst marketers are tricksters. They use the incredible
power of promotion, of advertising, and of storytelling to get us to
do something that's not in our long-term interest. It's good for
them, sure, but if we knew what they know, we probably wouldn't
play along.

How much should a diamond ring cost? Well, the diligent, hardworking diamond marketers spent forty years and almost $1 bil-
lion to persuade young men and their fiancées that it ought to cost
a lot more than makes sense.

And are cigarettes safe, sexy, and healthy? If you look at the TV
ads of the 1960s, it's sure easy to come to that conclusion. When
cigarettes finally fell, they fell hard. We don't like being tricked.

Diamonds are mere decoration, a one-time purchase. Smoking
is a habit, but a lot of people figured out how to wean themselves
from the addiction. Meat, on the other hand, is a very profitable,
very selfish, and dangerous method of feeding ourselves, one with
significant side effects that impact everyone.

Meat is also brilliantly marketed.

Think about it: We have almost no idea how it's made. Almost no
images of the supply chain (in some states, it's actually against the
law to videotape the process, even on public land).

Since you were born, McDonald's has spent more than $1 billion
advertising the connection between family, fun, and hamburgers.

And of course, Chicken McNuggets are not merely little scraps of reconstituted, breaded fried bits of scrap chicken, they're fun in a box.

Don't forget the Oscar Mayer Weinermobile. No kid cries when dad says he has to eat a hot dog.

Supermarkets use beef as a reliable profit center. It's easy to sell, it keeps longer than vegetables, and you can sell quite a bit of it.

Most of all, American culture has put the idea of meat at the center of our social experience. Of course there's meat on the menu. Of course they serve it on the airplane. Of course that's what you get at a catered event. It's sure to please, travels well, and it is almost impossible to prepare it terribly.

This story doesn't have to be true, and this story isn't an accident. Of course it happened on purpose.

The amount of meat consumed every year by the typical American is up nearly 50 percent in my lifetime. There are very few products this old that have experienced 50 percent growth over time. We're not drinking 50 percent more water or eating 50 percent more bread. We're not buying 50 percent more socks or using 50 percent more toothpaste. Nope, something else is at work here.

The food pyramid, propaganda served as truth in boring classrooms across the land, was a deliberate marketing effort, one that put meat at the base of the healthy diet.

As we eat more meals out of home, restaurant food becomes a bigger part of what we eat, and restaurants want food that's easy to sell, easy to prepare, easy to store, and high in profit. Again, the meat industry has figured out how to sell this to restaurants, and the restaurants, in turn, to us.

Meat is marketed as the elemental food for the rich (see steak houses) and the time-saving and protein-rich choice for the poor as well. A difficult balancing act, beautifully done.

The thing about cultural preference is that it is invisible. We don't say that we wear perfume because it is a cultural imperative, we actually think it makes us smell better. We don't say that we don't like to eat crickets because we didn't grow up with them, we say it's because they're "gross." And on and on.

And so, some people reading this will say that they order meat because it tastes better or because the human metabolism is designed to eat it. But, for more than half the people on the planet, those statements aren't true. No, it's culture that drives us to do this, and culture that drives our preferences.

Will this book change our culture, will it undermine the marketing behemoth? Almost certainly not, just as the surgeon general's report didn't end smoking.

So what will make the difference?

A simple one-word question. A countermarketing effort, one person to another, hand to hand, day to day.

"Really?"

As in, "You're *really* going to order that?"

"You're *really* going to eat that?"

"You've *really* got this on the menu?"

It takes very few upset people to undermine a brilliant marketing campaign. It takes just a few peers voicing their disapproval before people take their cigarettes outside or stop making racist jokes or join a new social network.

This is marketing too. Bottom-up marketing. Except we're not the bottom, we're merely people who care. We can market the idea that, just for today, eat something else. For yourself, for those around you.

Old habits die hard, but culture changes every day.

Just in time.

LESS MEAT; MORE DOUGH

▉ Paul Shapiro

Vice president, policy, The Humane Society of the United States

Many of us must save up to be able to take a holiday. We deprive ourselves in the short term, thinking about all the fun ways we'll be able to spend that hard-earned cash in the future. Yet there's one kind of holiday that can help break up the monotony of daily life while also saving us money. Taking occasional holidays from meat will actually save us dough. And indeed, many Americans across the country are already doing just that. We Americans now eat about 10 percent less meat per capita than we did in 2007. It seems that dietary concepts like the Three R's ("reducing" or "replacing" consumption of animal products while "refining" our diets) may finally be here to stay.

Some of this reduction may come from following popular movements like Meatless Mondays or Mark Bittman's Vegan Before 6 program. But, of course, there are many reasons so many of us are taking breaks from a meat-heavy diet. Wanting to look and feel better, to protect animals, and to help save the planet are just a few motives people commonly offer. But an additional benefit of keeping more animals off our plates is that it helps us keep more money in our wallets.

Meat, eggs, and dairy are costly and they're getting even more expensive. It's no secret that vegetarian foods are far less resource-intensive than the breeding and slaughtering of animals. That's one reason that—even with distorting federal handouts to the meat industry—meat-free options are often more affordable. For example, it's always cheaper to opt for Chipotle's bean and rice burritos—or its new chili-rubbed tofu sofritas—than the chain's meat options. Burger King's veggie burger will leave more bling in your bank account than a Whopper. And every single vegetarian entrée at P. F. Chang's is cheaper than every meat-based entrée the popular restaurant offers.

Of course, while saving money is a compelling reason to eat a little bit lower on the food chain, the more affordable options are also generally the ones that are better for us as well as for the planet. Prestigious public health organizations agree. As the American Institute for Cancer Research noted recently, "The research shows one thing very clearly: we all need to eat more plants and less meat."

Now that Americans are starting to take occasional holidays from meat, even factory farm interests are beginning to pay attention. You know our diets are shifting for the better when companies like Walmart start encouraging a reduction in meat consumption, and local Dollar Tree stores sell Hampton Creek's egg-free, plant-based mayo—a product that once might have been consigned solely to health food stores. In fact, if you don't happen to read the industry magazine *Meat+Poultry*, you may have missed its recent editorial asking meat producers, "Why doesn't the industry make meat analogs?" The writer notes that "Meat analogs are evolving and tasting better than ever" and quotes a meat scientist talking about companies like Tofurky, counseling, "Don't fight them, join them."

Indeed, that's already what's happening. Food giant Kraft may own Oscar Mayer, but it also owns Boca Burger. Kellogg's owns MorningStar Farms. Meat-centric diner chains like Johnny Rockets and Friendly's are now offering vegan burgers. Even Burger King—the king of burgers—is promoting Meatless Mondays.

The world is indeed shifting, and for the better. Pork giant Hormel recently bought another type of plant protein product: Skippy peanut butter. One benefit of this acquisition—according to another meat industry trade publication, *Meatingplace*—is that "activists are not using hidden cameras to scope out peanut abuse by Hormel's suppliers." Certainly not.

So many Americans are cutting down on meat consumption in fact that NASDAQ published a post looking at how "the death of meat" could impact your stock portfolio. The article concluded that investors should "think twice about holding long positions in meat industry stocks or exchange-traded securities" because "meat consumption has been steadily declining, which could play out into a huge profit potential."

It's always a good time to start new positive habits. But with meat prices projected to keep rising, there's never been a better time to start. Each time we sit down to eat, our choices can help make the world a better place. It's striking and exciting that something as simple as opting for hearty three-bean chili or pasta primavera instead of a drumstick or sausage can have such significant impact.

Holidays from meat are a win for our bodies, which will likely be lighter—literally. They're a win for our planet, since the burden we place on it will also be lighter. And they're a win for animals, which should make our consciences lighter. In fact, the only things that won't be lighter will be our wallets. Now that's the kind of break we could all use more often.

A NUDGE IN THE RIGHT DIRECTION

▍ Per Espen Stoknes

Author of *What We Think About When We Try Not to Think About Global Warming: Toward a New Psychology of Climate Action*

▍ Bradley Swain

Behavioral Researcher at the Common Cents Lab

Imagine for a moment that you are having a dinner party. You've spent most of the day shopping for food, cleaning your house, and cooking for your guests. As people trickle in and the drinks get poured, you put out a large bowl of potato chips for people to snack on, as a good host should. More people arrive and the chips are dwindling. As you go to refill the bowl, your friends cry, "Stop! Don't refill that bowl! Take it away, it's going to spoil my appetite."

Most people recognize what is going on here. Your friend is hoping you will remove the temptation of the chips. That makes sense on a human level, but to an economist the behavior is somewhat odd. Economic theory holds that choice is good but even more choices is better. Surely having the choice of eating potato chips is better than no choice, right? The problem is regular humans don't always act as economists think they should. Sometimes they need a nudge to help them make the best decision. A nudge, according to Richard Thaler and Cass Sunstein—two authors who coined the term in their 2008 book *Nudge: Improving Decisions about Health, Wealth, and Happiness*—is "any aspect of the choice architecture that alters people's behavior in a predictable way, without forbidding any options or significantly changing their economic incentives." Nudges may not be a silver bullet for society's meat consumption problem, but it is clear they can be a powerful tool for activists, educators and policy makers attempting to convince a meat-eating public to change their ways.

For decades classical economics was often the sole social science allowed at the policy table. With its sophisticated mathematical models and precise predictions, economics was treated as a sort of social physics. But if the assumptions of economics are correct, nudging shouldn't work. And yet, not everyone agrees. The study of nudges stems from the same common ancestral observation exemplified by the chip bowl conundrum: Human beings do not always behave according to rational self-interest. This may not be a surprising observation to anyone who has ever interacted with humans before. Still, the assumption that all humans make rational economic choices lies at the core of all traditional economic models.

Among the first academics to suggest people are not as rational as economists presume were Daniel Kahneman and Amos Tversky. Along with their graduate students Paul Slovic and Baruch Fischhoff, Kahneman and Tversky outlined a number of thought experiments demonstrating that humans not only deviate from the predictions made by classical economics but do so in predictable ways. They called these findings *heuristics* and *biases*. A heuristic is essentially academic jargon for a mental rule of thumb, while a bias is an inclination toward a particular view or outcome.

One example of a heuristic is called the *anchoring heuristic*. Anchoring is the tendency to rely too heavily on the first piece of information offered (the anchor). It is interesting that this includes arbitrary information. To demonstrate, imagine I give you a list of items that I will be auctioning off: a bottle of wine, a new MP3 player, and some chocolate among other items of similar value. Then I tell you to write down the last two digits of your social security number next to the wine, the last two digits of your telephone number next to the MP3 player, and the last two digits of your zip code next to the chocolate. After promising that I am not trying to steal your identity, I ask you to bid on the items. How much do you think these seemingly arbitrary numbers will influence the price you are willing to pay? Most people think the arbitrary numbers won't influence them. But when a similar experiment was conducted in a lab at MIT, researchers found that in fact, people's bids varied significantly. Participants with low two-digit numbers bid substantially less on the item, while people with high numbers bid substantially more. Even though the participants knew the numbers were arbitrary, the number still acted as an anchor, causing them to adjust the price they were willing to pay.

These findings and others suggest that most people do not walk around with a fixed set of preferences in their heads as economists previously theorized. Rather, our preferences are constructed in the moment. We use salient reference points to make up our preferences on the fly.

The theory of defaults can teach us a little more about how we construct preferences. Consider the following: In the late 1990s, the Dutch Ministry of Health, Welfare and Sport found itself struggling to find citizens willing to donate their organs for transplant. Even after a multimillion-dollar advertising campaign, the country could convince only 27 percent of its population to register as organ donors. At the same time, the UK and Germany were facing a similar organ deficit, with between 10 and 12 percent of their populations willing to be donors. What was particularly frustrating to the Dutch ministry was the fact that many of their culturally similar neighbors, such as Austria and Sweden, boasted impressive rates of organ donation hovering close to 98 percent. How could countries so similar display such a disparity?

The answer lies in the way a single question on a government form was phrased. Two researchers from Columbia University realized that when faced with a difficult choice, people often take the path of least resistance, meaning they take no action. In the Netherlands, UK, and Germany, the form asks people to check a box if they want to be an organ donor. In the case of these three countries, the default option was effectively the choice not to be a donor. In Sweden and Austria, on the other hand, the form asks people to check if they don't want to be an organ donor. The easiest choice is still not checking the box, but the default is to register. Countries that set organ donation as the default netted 71 percent more organ donors.[1]

Many of the tools outlined have implications for anyone who wishes to change how much meat people eat, but so far we have only tantalizing initial results on how the findings could be specifically applied. Take once again the example of the chips: If a simple nudge like creating a room's distance between you and the bag is enough to make you stop eating them, how might be we design similar nudges to make people eat less meat?

One interesting example comes from a team led by Brian Wansink at Cornell University. Wansink ran an experiment using "magic" soup bowls. The researchers wanted to see if simply creating visual cues, much like taking the chip bowl out of direct sight, would result in people eating less. Experimenters recruited hungry participants who were then divided into two groups. Both groups were asked to sit and eat soup until they were full. The twist was that one group had bowls with secret tubes attached to the bottom. These tubes slowly refilled participants' soup as they ate. Participants in the second group had to ask the experimenter to refill their bowl if they wanted more. The researchers found that participants whose bowls "magically" stayed full ate on average 73 percent more soup than those who had to refill their bowl by request.[2] It was surprising that the participants whose bowls were continually refilled reported feeling less full than participants who had to ask for more soup.

Health conscious business and cafeteria managers should take note. Providing larger cups, plates, and bowls does encourage cus-tomers to eat more of whatever you put in them, but diners might not even be happy about it. Might we be able to reduce meat con-sumption by 10 percent by simply reducing the size of plates by 10 percent?

Another study by Wansink investigated how food options, even when they aren't necessarily chosen, affect meal outcomes. Wan-sink found that just ensuring certain nutritious foods, such as green beans or bananas, were more easily available than other foods helped people make healthier food choices, even if they didn't consciously choose to eat green beans or bananas. Similarly, mak-ing fried potatoes and meat visible caused people to take larger portions of unhealthy food, even if they didn't consciously prefer the potatoes or meat.

Semantics, too, can be incredibly important tools in the nudge architects' toolbox. We see this clearly in a study conducted at a res-taurant in Oslo that looked at the effect of simply renaming the "vegetarian options." The restaurant rebranded vegetable-based menu items with fancier names like "Mexican-style taco" and made vegetarian options the special dish of the day. As a result of these tweaks, customers at the restaurant ended up eating meat less fre-quently. The change was seen particularly among customers who did not have a strong connection to nature.

Similarly, varying descriptions of the same problem can lead to systematically different decisions. This is sometimes known as *framing*. Psychologist Irwin Levin demonstrated one of the earliest exam-ples of framing when he asked people in two different groups how they felt about either buying 75 percent lean meat or buying 25 per-cent fat meat. The people in the 75 percent lean group described the experience much more positively than those in the 25 percent fat group, even though logically these two descriptions are the same.[3] Other studies have shown that reframing the wording of a politically charged product is effective—for example, more consumers volun-tarily purchased a flight with a carbon offset than a flight with a car-bon tax. Might a similar idea work for reducing meat consumption?

The research is pretty clear: When combined with traditional methods of education and persuasion, a nudge in the right direc-tion can tip the scales on important issues. Actions, particularly our own and those of significant others, can speak louder than facts and words, creating a virtuous circle. Behavior influences attitudes that grow into public support for greener policies. With public support, the policies can be strengthened to shape behaviors and attitudes in even more climate-friendly ways. And the cycle continues.

THE FUTURE OF FOOD

Josh Balk

Vice president, farm animal protection, The Humane Society of the United States; co-founder of Hampton Creek

Today, we are witnessing the slow but steady dismantling of U.S. factory farming right before our very eyes. As of November 2016, eleven states have banned formerly standard practices that were used to cruelly and inhumanely confine egg-laying chickens, calves, and mother pigs inside small cages. Many other major food companies have taken steps to phase out similarly abusive conditions.

But while the changes being made from within the farm industry are important, industrial animal agribusiness is feeling the pressure from outside influences as well. This pressure is being applied in the form of restaurant menu changes, new product lines, and even start-up companies. Taken together, these developments signal the beginning of the end for what is perhaps the most extensive exploitation of animals the world has ever known.

When I decided to become vegan fourteen years ago, the number of food options available at both grocery stores and restaurants was disappointedly limited. I was forced to shop at natural food stores (forget about mainstream retailers carrying vegan fare) and restaurant menus proved similarly disappointing. I stuck with it because of my concern for animals, but I can see why people hesitate when thinking about changing up their eating habits. To some, it simply doesn't seem worth the inconvenience. Fast-forward to 2016, and times have dramatically changed. Chipotle now offers tofu-based sofritas. Subway is promoting its falafel and vegan patty selections. White Castle made its veggie slider a permanent fixture on its menu. And at the grocery store, every major chain from Walmart to Costco to Safeway offers hordes of plant-based meats.

The growth of plant-based foods runs parallel to the reduced consumption of animal products. In fact, fewer land animals are being raised and killed for food today than in 2007, despite the fact that our country's population has increased. That's because while more people are switching to animal products raised in more humane conditions (like cage-free eggs), they're also reducing their overall consumption of meat and replacing animal-based foods with those from plants.

One of the driving forces behind this transformation of the food system comes from an unlikely quarter: Silicon Valley. Peter Thiel, one of the co-founders of PayPal, is a leader of innovative food options. Bill Gates and Li Ka-shing, the wealthiest person in Asia, are as well. So are Marc Benioff, the wealthiest person in San Francisco; Vinod Khosla, the founder of the internationally renowned firm Khosla Ventures; Eduardo Saverin, a co-founder of Facebook; and Uni-President Enterprises Corporation, one of the largest food conglomerates in Asia. All told, more than a dozen billionaires and the multibillion-dollar firms with which they are associated have invested in start-up companies working to create non-animal-based foods. These companies use plants, which are less expensive, more sustainable, and have a higher nutrient profile than their animal counterparts, to create food items that are both sustainable and tasty. More than 90 percent of the world's plants have never been explored as food options, meaning there's a vast universe of untapped potential for companies to utilize.

One of these companies is Impossible Foods, which is using science to create plant-based burgers. The founder, Pat Brown, discovered that much of the flavor in a hamburger comes from an iron-containing

compound called heme, most commonly found in blood, which inter-
acts with various molecules within the patty. Brown has found that
plants can duplicate heme's qualities, thus creating a burger that
smells and tastes just like a backyard barbecue.

Beyond Meat, another plant-based meat company, uses a process called extrusion to create its products. If you've ever pulled
apart a piece of chicken meat, you may have noticed the way it's
composed in sections of strings. For decades, vegetarian meats
were created by blending together plant proteins; the resulting
meat substitute had a consistency very different from animal flesh.
However, by using an extruder, Beyond Meat products is attempting to mimic the texture of chicken meat.

On the dairy side, a company called Perfect Day is creating
animal-free milk through a method similar to how microbreweries
make beer. Milk is made up of proteins, fats, calcium, potassium,
sugars, and other components. Perfect Day's proteins come from
yeast, and the other ingredients come from vegetables. Once combined together, the ingredients form a synthetic milk product that
bypasses the cow altogether. As a bonus, it's designed to be dramatically healthier than traditional milk and is produced with a lighter
carbon footprint.

On the even more experimental side, a company called Modern
Meadow is working to duplicate animal cells to form muscles. These
could then potentially be turned into meat, all without slaughtering a live animal. While many years away from a commercial food
product, the company is much closer to debuting a line of leather
goods. The leather is being created using *in vitro* technology, which
is simpler than the process used to create flesh and does not require
the same level of FDA approval. (However, some lucky people have
already eaten prototypes of Modern Meadow's meat products, and
I hear the reviews have been quite favorable.)

It's important to remember that these innovative companies are
possible today in part because of the efforts of trailblazers like Tofurky, Field Roast, and Gardein. For years, these pioneers have
demonstrated that plant-based food does not have to be restricted
to salads and grilled vegetable platters.

Ultimately, the trajectory couldn't be clearer. As a society, we're
finally realizing the harmful effects of eating vast amounts of meat,

eggs, and dairy. This diet isn't good for our health, for the planet, or for animals. It seems clear that we've reached an important turning point—as we move into the middle of the twenty-first century, our food system will likely never be the same again.

THE MORAL ARC OF ANIMAL RIGHTS

Michael Shermer

Author of *The Moral Arc: How Science Makes Us Better People*

> *When I view all beings not as special creations, but as the lineal descendants of some few beings which lived long before the first bed of the Cambrian system was deposited, they seem to me to become ennobled.*
>
> —CHARLES DARWIN, ON THE ORIGIN OF SPECIES, 1859

Darwin's observation lays the foundation for a moral starting point grounded in evolutionary theory. In my 2015 book, *The Moral Arc: How Science and Reason Lead Humanity Toward Truth, Justice, and Freedom*, my moral starting point is the survival and flourishing of sentient beings. By *survival* I mean "the instinct to live," and by *flourishing* I mean "having adequate sustenance, safety, shelter, and social relations for physical and mental health." By *sentient* I mean "emotive, perceptive, sensitive, responsive, conscious, and especially the capacity to feel and to suffer." Instead of using criteria such as tool use, language, reasoning, or intelligence, I go deeper into our evolved brains toward these more basic emotive capacities. There is sound science behind this proposition.

According to the Cambridge Declaration on Consciousness—a statement issued in 2012 by an international group of prominent cognitive neuroscientists, neuropharmacologists, neuroanatomists, and computational neuroscientists—there is a continuity between humans and most other higher order nonhuman animals, and sentience is the most important common characteristic. The neural pathways of emotions, for example, are not confined to higher-level cortical structures in the brain, but are found in evolutionarily older subcortical regions. Artificially stimulating the same regions in human and nonhuman animal brains produces the same emotional reactions in both. Attentiveness, decision making, and the emotional capacity to feel and suffer are found across the branches of the evolutionary tree. This is what brings all humans and many nonhuman animals into our moral sphere.

If we are going to take seriously the moral precept of the right of all sentient beings to survive and flourish, and if we are going to continue to push the arc of the moral universe toward justice and freedom and expand the moral sphere to include more and more sentient beings, then we should show the courage of our convictions by acting on our beliefs. When? Here I can relate to the prayer of Saint Augustine of Hippo, who, when a young man, struggled with sexual passions he knew he should resist, cried out to the Lord, "Grant me chastity and continence, but not yet." Still, I am moved by the words of Victor Hugo when he wrote, "Nothing is more powerful than an idea whose time has come." I can think of no reason why now is not the time for sentient beings to be granted rights. But which sentient beings and which rights?

For wild species, this is nothing more than allowing them the freedom to hunt and forage for food in their natural environment and to protect them from poachers and the excessive encroachment of civilization into their habitats. For domesticated species, I believe this means ending factory farming and shifting toward family farming— giving domesticated animals a more humane version of the environment in which they survived and flourished for the past 10,000 years before the advent of factory farming in the twentieth century. Our human ancestors made a tacit bargain with the wild animals they domesticated—they gave us their eggs, milk, fur, and flesh in exchange for food and water and protection from predators so that they could survive and reproduce and flourish—and so we have a moral duty to maintain our end of the deal if we intend to continue the taking.

In *The Moral Arc* I outline a "Provisional Ten Commandments" based on reason and science, which I then attempt to apply to the treatment of animals. The first two commandments—the Golden-Rule Principle and the Ask-First Principle, might apply to animal rights by asking ourselves how our actions in regard to other species affect their capacity to survive and flourish. We can imagine how we might feel if we were, say, a chimpanzee locked up in a cold steel cage injected with human diseases. We might visualize ourselves as dolphins frolicking about a cove when all of a sudden a machete cuts through the water and slashes us open to bleed to death. Or we might picture being a steer, taking our final walk down our own green mile, hearing our comrades falling one by one.

In so identifying with other species and taking their perspective, we might find a way to apply the Happiness Principle and the Liberty Principle, in which we should never seek happiness and liberty when it leads to the unhappiness and loss of liberty of another sentient being. We might also consider the Fairness Principle, based on John Rawls's concepts of the "veil of ignorance" and the "original position," in which we are ignorant of our position in society when determining rules and laws that affect everyone, so imagine this applied to ourselves as sentient beings not knowing if we would be born as a farmer or a farm animal. Given what we know, which farm would be fairest, a family farm or a factory farm? The question answers itself.

Continuing through the Provisional Ten Commandments, the Reason Principle would imply that we should reason our way toward rational choices about the foods we eat and the animals we use (for hunting, recreation, or pets), opting when possible for food products from companies that consider animal welfare and the environment, or hunting organizations like Ducks Unlimited that aim for species conservation, or pets from rescue shelters instead of pet mills. The Defend Others Principle applies not only to children, the mentally ill, the old, and the handicapped but also to domesticated animals, especially because we purposefully bred out of them their natural capacity for surviving on their own in the wild. Finally, The Biophilia Principle would apply to all plants and animals, along with the air and water, in terms of creating a sustainable environment for untold generations of human and nonhuman animals still to come.

To further this moral progress, from the bottom up we can vote with our voices and our dollars for the type of food we want and push the market toward this more moral stance. And from the top down we can work for legislation that abolishes the exploitation of sentient beings, expanding our moral sphere to include the great apes and marine mammals and working our way down the many branches and twigs of the evolutionary tree that Charles Darwin so eloquently described in the final sentence of *On the Origin of Species*:

> There is grandeur in this view of life, with its several powers, having been originally breathed into a few forms or into one; and that, whilst this planet has gone cycling on according to the fixed law of gravity, from so simple a beginning endless forms most beautiful and most wonderful have been, and are being, evolved.

HE WON'T REDUCE HIS MEAT EATING!

Susan Page

Author of *If I'm So Wonderful, Why Am I Still Single?* and *Why Talking Is Not Enough*

If you are living—and cooking—together with someone who does not share your values about reducing the meat in your diet, this can create tension and even "fights" in your relationship. Whether you are the one who thinks reducing your meat intake is simply too hard to do, or even silly, or you seriously want your partner to stop eating so much meat, this difference can cause great strife between you. What can you do about it?

For the purposes of this example, let's assume that you want to be a reducetarian and that your partner is a man and loves meat!

But of course meat-eating preferences can go in any gender direction. Substitute the pronouns that suit your situation. Also, remember you may apply the same strategies I suggest here to other problems in your relationship.

So he is entrenched in meat eating and just won't stop. He loves his steaks, his sausages, and his chicken tacos! This drives you crazy. You know how harmful this is to his health and to the planet! You fight about it to no avail.

Here's the solution to the problem: Stop trying to change him.

It's true: He is the one creating the problem by refusing to change his meat habit. But realize this: You are the one who is creating the upset in the relationship by continuing to bring it up and making an issue out of it. What is more important to you: a harmonious atmosphere in your home or getting him to stop eating so much meat? You can "solve this problem" all by yourself by accepting your partner's position, in a spirit of love and goodwill, and letting it be okay.

The loving acceptance I am talking about here is very different from "giving in." When you were fighting about meat, you had no choice but to "give in," grudgingly, feeling you were losing a battle, feeling powerless and upset. When you make the inner shift to loving acceptance, suddenly now, you have taken your own power back. Your personal happiness no longer depends on something your partner does or does not do! You were giving him all the power over your own happiness.

When you lovingly accept your partner's meat eating, it is no longer a problem; it is a fact of life. A problem has to be *solved*. A fact of life needs to be *adapted to*, in a mature way that relieves the most upset for the most people. You are not solving the problem of his meat eating but outgrowing it by developing a new level of consciousness, by committing yourself to a higher goal: discovering a larger you who can singlehandedly create a happier relationship for both of you.

Of course, it is true that your partner "should" cooperate and work on changing his meat habit. It is a fact that eating too much meat is bad for his health and for the planet. You are absolutely right and fair about what you are asking for. Also, you have probably worked on communicating your desire to him in tactful ways, using the best communication skills you have. You are right! He is wrong to keep upsetting you and destroying his health!

But being right is the booby prize in a relationship! You get to be right, but you don't get to feel closer to your partner. You don't create an atmosphere in which he feels closer to you. You don't get to solve the problem. You don't create a warm, loving home. You don't obtain any of the BIG prizes! All you get is this tiny booby prize, you get to be right and make him wrong. But when you continue to insist on being right, the problem is still there, and you are still unhappy. And so is he.

Trust me when I tell you, it's not worth it. Go for the big prizes! You can do this by yourself, without waiting for your partner to cooperate or not cooperate! If you can quietly, graciously be the "big" person here, and let go of your need for him to eat less meat, all of a sudden, with just a slight inner shift on your part, the problem is gone, you feel more control because you no longer depend on him to change for you to feel happy, and he is going to be grateful that you have let go of harping at him about this issue. Think of your gracious acceptance as a loving gift you give him. He gets to be who he is without someone he is close to criticizing him all the time.

Loving acceptance will require work on your part! It will require discipline and commitment. You will have to use great restraint. You'll have to practice and fail a few times. Sometimes you will have to act as if you feel loving, even though inside you are angry. There is no rule that says you always have to act exactly the way you feel. You can't change how you feel. But you do have control over how you behave, and it is slight changes in your behavior, even when you feel different inside, that will make a major difference in the harmony in your home. It won't be easy. But think of it as providing a higher consciousness in your relationship. You don't have to talk about your decision to change to loving acceptance. Just do it, as an experiment. See what an impact your higher consciousness has on your family. If you are the cook in the family, you may even have to continue cooking meat for your partner, as a gesture of goodwill, of love, of acceptance. But if you care about your relationship, this is the only pathway for you. Just let go!

Change happens in an atmosphere of love and acceptance. The more you badger your partner, the more he will resist and become defensive. It is appropriate for him to defend who he is and what he thinks and likes!

If you back off, and quietly continue the eating habits that suit you, you may be surprised at the gradual change that might take place in your partner. That is the only way the change will happen, and it is the only way for you to be a truly loving, respectful partner.

Spiritual writer Thomas Moore says, "A slight shift in consciousness has more impact on living than major efforts at change." I'm sure your effort to get your partner to change by eating less meat has been major. You have harped and nagged, made your "I" statements, communicated your needs, been sweet about it, gotten angry about it, made him wrong, felt utterly frustrated, carried on with your girlfriends about it, and generally made it into a big problem that never got solved. But a "slight shift in consciousness," when you realize that a big part of love is acceptance, will have a major impact on your life—in more ways than you can imagine before you try it.

Breathe. Take back your power by making loving acceptance your goal and by being really good at it! Ride the horse in the direction it is already going. Stop trying to control the world and make it into exactly what you wish it were. Surrender to what is, as a deliberate, intentional strategy. You will feel great inner strength, and when your partner sees the shift in you and feels your new inner strength, he may start moving in your direction.

BEYOND CARNISM

Melanie Joy

Author of *Why We Love Dogs, Eat Pigs, and Wear Cows: An Introduction to Carnism*

Today, many of us are aware that eating less meat is good for our health, for animals, and for the environment. What most people don't realize, though, is that eating less meat can actually be good for our minds—that reducing the amount of meat we eat can actually increase our psychological and emotional well-being.

As a psychologist, my interest has been on how certain food choices impact us psychologically—and on what this means for ourselves and our world. My research, corroborated by others, has found that eating meat, eggs, and dairy requires us to diminish the very qualities that are fundamental to our psychological and emotional well-being. When we eat animal products, we disconnect from our authentic thoughts and dampen our natural empathy; our logic becomes compromised and our emotions become numbed. The result is that we act against our deeper values, values such as compassion and justice. And all this happens automatically and unconsciously.

For example, when we bite into a juicy steak, we think of it as a tasty piece of food and feel pleasure. Yet if someone informed us that the meat was actually from a golden retriever, we would likely no longer think of it as a juicy piece of food, but as a bloody part of a dead animal. And our pleasure would turn to disgust. This latter response is our authentic response; most of us naturally empathize with animals and don't want to harm them. We have simply been conditioned to block this authentic response when it comes to the animals we have learned to classify as edible.

Most of us recognize that all animals feel pleasure and pain, yet we rarely, if ever, question why we treat different types of animals so differently—some we love, and others we slaughter. We have developed a pattern of behavior that causes extensive harm to ourselves and others, and yet this pattern remains unquestioned because it is largely invisible. But there is a way to break this pattern. First, we need to understand its root cause.

What my research uncovered is that there is an invisible belief system that conditions us to eat certain animals. I named this system carnism; carnism is essentially the opposite of veganism. Most of us believe that only vegans and vegetarians follow a belief system. However, in meat-eating cultures around the world—though the type of species consumed changes—people learn to classify only a small handful of animals as edible. All the rest are inedible and often "disgusting." When eating animals is not a necessity, which is the case for many people today, then it is a choice—and choices always stem from beliefs.

Carnism is a dominant belief system, meaning that it is invisible, and it is woven through the very structure of society to shape norms, laws, beliefs, behaviors, etc. For example, when we study nutrition, we actually study carnistic nutrition—but we don't realize it because carnistic bias is so deeply embedded in society. Carnism is a violent system; meat cannot be procured without violence (and egg and dairy production also cause extensive harm to animals).

Carnism requires us to support a practice that is actually counter to our core values; most of us care about animals and don't want them to suffer, especially when that suffering is unnecessary. We value compassion and justice. So carnism (like other violent systems) uses a set of defense mechanisms that distort our thoughts and numb our feelings so that we act against our values without fully realizing what we are doing. Carnism teaches us how not to think and feel.

For instance, carnism teaches us to think of farmed animals as abstractions, as lacking any individuality or personality of their own: a pig is a pig, and all pigs are the same. This distorted thinking distances us from our natural ability to identify and empathize with these beings; it is often distressing for people to consider eating a pig whom they've gotten to know personally. And carnism teaches us to see farmed animals as objects; it is far easier to eat something, than someone, to eat a piece of livestock rather than a living being. And carnism teaches us to suspend our logic and accept the myths of meat as the facts of meat—to believe in what I refer to as the Three Ns of Justification: eating animals is normal, natural, and necessary. Such myths are, of course, nothing new; consider how they have been used to justify slavery, male dominance, and heterosexual supremacy.

The good news is that when we start reducing our consumption of meat (and eggs and dairy) we stop reinforcing the logical distortions and emotional numbing that carnism engenders. So, when we reduce our consumption of carnistic products, we reduce our need for carnistic defenses, which increases our psychological and emotional well-being. And we are therefore better able to make choices that reflect and reinforce what we authentically think and feel, rather than what we have been taught to think and feel.

SIMPLE STRATEGIES FOR SUCCESS

Terra Wellington

Author of *The Mom's Guide to Growing Your Family Green: Saving the Earth Begins at Home*

Several years ago our family was the typical American, eat-meat-every-day family. We ate meat even when there was sufficient plant protein already on the table. It seemed like a cultural imperative, and as parents, we were raised that way. Over the past several years, however, we have changed how we eat, including reducing our meat consumption and adding more veggies and fruits to our diet. I've become a full vegetarian, while the rest of my family is more comfortable living a more flexible reducetarian lifestyle. We made the change for many reasons, both in terms of our personal health and the health of the planet.

If your family is looking to make a similar change, there are a few simple tips we've picked up along the way that may help. It takes equal parts vision, knowledge, and strategy to make a successful transition. Remember, this isn't simply a food transition; it's a different way of thinking about food entirely.

The following is some practical advice that may also help you find joy during the process.

DON'T MAKE A BIG DEAL ABOUT IT

Without a cultural background of reducing meat consumption, the best strategy is to not make a big deal about it. Save yourself a lot of stress and don't make a big announcement about the change; this will only open yourself up to a lot of questioning and self-doubt. Every plate will be analyzed. Rather than starting out with a bang, approach the food change incrementally, thoughtfully—and tastily. Later, you can start talking more about the reasoning and even get into nutrition education and label reading if you want to (there's actually a lot of nerdy stuff involved that can be quite empowering).

START WITH MONDAYS

Start small, just one day a week. The Meatless Monday program is a great campaign to join. Maybe you'll take it further as the months and years progress, adding on more meatless days as you feel more and more comfortable. But one day a week is a doable commitment from the beginning.

FOCUS ON DELICIOUS MEALS

Instead of pointing out what's missing (the meat) at the dinner table, center food conversation around exciting new recipes. Try new side dishes and new entrees. This makes the journey a food adventure instead of a loss. Ask for feedback if you feel comfortable and get the family involved in the cooking process. Make it all as natural as possible. How your family responds to the new tastes will also help you tweak the menu going forward.

REALIZE THERE IS A TASTE SHIFT

Our brains are programmed to habitually want what they are fed, especially if it tastes good. But food is not just about taste; it's also tied up in our emotional and cultural relationships and traditions.

If you are used to eating tasty meat-filled meals as a family, the brain will likely associate certain foods with great taste and also a loving environment. Introducing new foods and new tastes is like making new memories and new connections—be aware that your brain may initially be tentative about them. It may take time to create a new comfort level. And that's okay.

SAMPLE WELL-PREPARED MEATLESS MEALS

When we first started reducing my family's meat consumption, it was really important to have a vision. Going to well-reviewed vegetarian restaurants or trying vegetarian meals at healthy boutique restaurants and farm-fresh events gave us insight into what was possible at home. There's so much inspiration to be found if you're looking for it. You can find resources all over the place: regional farmer events, farmers' markets, co-op grocery stores' announcement boards, the slow food movement, HappyCow.net, vegetarian restaurant review sites, and even your friends.

INCREASE YOUR VEGGIES AND FRUITS

Around the same time we started to reduce our meat consumption, we also began increasing our veggie and fruit consumption across the board. We displayed much of our fresh fruits on beautiful vintage platters and bowls on the kitchen counter—so tempting! And we were constantly looking for interesting ways to get veggies into all our meals—steamed, cut up raw, put into diverse salads or transformed into delicious sides. Remember, presentation counts. We discovered that the farmers' market food tasted way better than what we found at the grocery store—most of it was organic or nearly organic. We also started growing an organic garden, which produced a delicious harvest of homegrown tomatoes. In addition, we joined a community-supported agriculture (CSA) program with a local farm cooperative. This subscription gave us a weekly box of seasonal veggies. It was always a box of surprises and included lots of veggies we hadn't ever tried before. In order to not waste the food, we had to learn about it and try it. As a result, over a couple of years we became much more adventurous and open to veggie possibilities. The kids would help us look up veggies on the Internet to figure out what they were and what to do with them.

All in all, the transition has been a big success so far. We eat more fresh food, more veggies and fruits, less meat, more organic, and very little junk food. Now, our children notice when people eat a lot of meat and not many veggies, but their brains and stomachs crave produce and fresher food. We hope that our new food culture will remain a positive example for our children as they get older. At the very least, we've given them a great start!

WHY WE CRAVE MEAT IN THE FIRST PLACE

■ Marta Zaraska

Author of *Meathooked: The History and Science of Our 2.5-Million-Year Obsession with Meat*

According to Gallup, in 1943 the number of Americans who didn't eat meat was about 2 percent. Then came the calls for ethical treatment of animals and studies on the adverse health effects of red meat consumption. So did we all rush to become vegetarians? Not really. Although by 2012 the number of people in United States who consider themselves vegetarian has risen to 5 percent (again according to Gallup), another survey showed that 60 percent of the American self-described vegetarians actually consume red meat, poultry or fish—at least occasionally.[1] Which brings us back to 2.4 percent of committed vegetarians—about the same as in 1943. The number of people who truly eschew meat in the United States is so low that the Faunalytics executive director Che Green went so far as to call vegans and vegetarians "a blip on the demographic radar."

On the other hand, we now know that giving up meat would be one of the simplest ways to lower the risk of dramatic climate changes. Of all greenhouse gases released by humans, 14.5 percent are down to our livestock. If this number doesn't seem that large, consider this: It's about the same as emissions from all of transportation combined: Passenger cars, trucks, ships, airplanes, etc. According to a recent report by the British think tank Chatham House, if we want to prevent catastrophic global warming, we need to curb our meat consumption.

If we stopped eating meat we would have more land and water to grow food and feed the planet. We would live longer (the vegetarian Seventh-day Adventists in California, for example, live on average 9.5 (men) and 6.1 (women) years longer than other Californians).[2] By saving over 70 billion animals worldwide from slaughter we would reduce suffering tremendously. And yet, the vast majority of people do not want to stop eating meat. Does meat give us something—chemically, nutritionally—that no other food can? Is our meat addiction cultural? Psychological? What does meat offer people that despite its costs—the guilt, the ruined arteries, the polluted planet—we keep eating it?

The question that has stayed unanswered far too long, while we keep arguing health and ethical aspects of meat consumption, is this: Why do we eat meat at all? The common answer many people give—"because I like it"—is not enough. It's a bit like a teenage girl telling her parents, who are anxious about an inappropriate boyfriend, that she's dating him "because I love him." At first glance, it seems like a good response. But she doesn't love the boy "just because." She loves this particular human male because his body gives off pheromones that attract her, because culturally she is predisposed to be drawn toward tall and muscular types, because she was raised by, say, a controlling mother and an insecure father, so she likes her boyfriends to be free-spirited. Same with meat. We don't eat it "just because we like it." There are many reasons meat is so attractive to us.

Our ancestors started eating meat about 2.5 million years ago, and—as some scientists say—that change in diet has actually made us human. Not only did meat eating help us migrate out of Africa but it was even behind our thinned hair and profuse sweating. Is that the reason we crave it so much? Do we simply have meat in our genes? Or maybe it's all about the taste of meat? Is it the 2-methyl-3-furanthiol or one of the other 1,000 volatile compounds that together make up the specific, mouth-watering scent of cooked meat? Is it the umami taste (Japanese for "delicious") that is found mostly in meat, mushrooms, and milk? Or maybe it's the skillful marketing and lobbying of the powerful meat industry, with its $186 billion in annual sales in the United States alone, that keeps us hooked on animal protein against our best interests? Or maybe we eat meat simply out of habit, because it got so engrained in our culture, religion, and history that we just cannot let go of it? Do we eat meat because over the centuries it came to symbolize masculinity, power over the poor, over nature, and over other nations? Is our love of meat a kind of addiction—psychological, chemical—or maybe both?

Just like it may be hard to stop drinking alcohol if you don't know why you got addicted in the first place, it may be hard to give up meat if you don't know why it is that you crave it. To successfully reduce our meat consumption, we should first become aware of meat's many meanings—only then can the hooks can be undone. The taste can be replaced by products containing meat's potent mixture of umami, fat, and the aromas created in the Maillard reaction (a chemical reaction between amino acids and reducing sugars that gives meat its desirable flavor). The protein hunger can be satisfied with lentils, beans, and even with peanut butter sandwiches. Government policies can be reversed, subsidies diverted, and meat tax introduced. We can take advantage of our psychological wiring and create positive associations for vegetarian meals by pairing them with foods we already love and by eating them at fun, social occasions. We should emphasize convenience and the price of plant-based diets, and not necessarily just their healthiness, because that's what people buy. We should try to change the image of meat substitutes by showing that is what many athletic, masculine men eat, and that "veg" can make you strong and beautiful. That is, after all, how meat has been sold to us for years.

I'm not saying we should all turn vegetarian tomorrow. Even though I do believe that in the future humanity will eat mostly plant-based foods, I also believe that pushing for dietary purity is not the way to go, and it may actually backfire—as it did a few times in the past. Instead, we should reward cutting down meat consumption—reducetarianism—whether it means cutting down by 10, by 20, or by 99 percent. We should stop flogging vegetarians who sometimes secretly eat meat. After all, compared to the Western average, they likely did manage to change their diets substantially. If you are an ethical vegetarian, think about it: What would save more lives—if one person stopped eating meat altogether, or if millions cut out just one meat-based meal a month?

What's most important, though, is to be aware of factors that drive our food choices, instead of blindly following our routines, our culture, the advertising. We shouldn't stick to our dietary habits only by default. We must analyze our relationship with meat, look deep into our biology and history to untangle the web of reasons meat is so hard to give up. That is the first step we need to take to unhook people from animal protein.

THE PORNOGRAPHY AND SEXUAL POLITICS OF EATING MEAT

Carol J. Adams

Author of *The Sexual Politics of Meat: A Feminist-Vegetarian Critical Theory*

In 1990, my book *The Sexual Politics of Meat* was published. Usually the phrase that follows is "to critical acclaim." In fact, full-page reviews challenging its thesis appeared around the world. The writers were confused and angry: How could "meat" have sexual politics attached to it? How could misogyny be expressed through what (or who) we eat?

The Sexual Politics of Meat begins by arguing that a link exists between meat eating and notions of masculinity and virility in the Western world. A belief exists that strength (male-identified) comes from eating "strong animals" (for instance, beef), and that men eating vegetables expresses passivity or femininity. Twenty-five years later means twenty-five years for examples to proliferate: various male-identified locations—such as steak houses, fraternities, strip clubs, and barbecues—offer masculine atmospheres promising both male bonding and meat. Fast-food hamburger companies like Burger King, Hardee's, and Carl's Jr. fall over each other trying to offer the raunchiest ad they can get on television. These ads always feature a slippage between the sexually posed women's bodies they feature and the oversize hamburger the woman is eating. Or menus might carry items like "Double D Cup Breast of Turkey Sandwich." Just who is being consumed?

Anti-tofu advertisements and comments turn on the link between meat eating and masculinity. In this worldview, to choose tofu is to be less of a man. Perhaps the most telling advertisement was not an ad for meat, but for beer: "Putting together a BBQ: +374 Man Points. Cooking tofu sausages on it: –417 Man Points."

It's not only human females who are the subject of these sexist depictions by the meat industry, but also nonhuman female animals. For example, magazines devoted to animal agriculture carry advertisements depicting female animals as sexy, busty, high heeled, and stockinged, with a "come hither" appearance. "Yes, make us pregnant," their cartoon images beg. "Yes, I want to give you one more piglet a year." One drug company placed a cow in the passenger seat of a fire truck, and asked, "What would she be doing if she weren't pregnant?" The implication: She would be taking a job from a fireman. Writes Chel Terrell for *Cattle Today*, "If a cow is not going to produce a calf every year, she's simply a freeloader."

It's not a surprise that females are depicted in such sexist ways given that female animals are at the heart of meat consumption, because it is their pregnancies in captivity that ensure the production of animals to be consumed. Consider the cow that must produce calves so that she continues to lactate, otherwise her freeloader status is confirmed. Her calf is taken from her shortly after birth, to ensure that her milk will go to human consumers. Both pregnant and lactating, her life span is four years, when she might have lived twenty.

Hostile terms for women such as cow, chick, sow, old biddy, and hen derive from such female beings who have absolutely no control over their reproductive choices. Their ability to be exploited lowers their standing and gives a powerful, negative charge to the meaning of the slang arising from their exploitation.

Misogyny, understood as a bias against or hatred of women, flourishes in meat-eating environments. Besides advertisements that link meat eating and masculinity, others depict animality and femaleness (women are shown animalized, animals feminized and sexualized): a full-bodied buxom pig, wearing heels, is "Moanin' for the Bone." A shrimp attired in a long pink dress coyly announcing she is "Shrimplee D'Elicious! Peel me & eat me." Like the female farmed animals depicted in the advertisements that I mentioned above, these female bodies want to be used.

The problem isn't the advertisements themselves, but the way in which they normalize dominant attitudes about consumption and sex roles. Discomforted by reminders of bleeding, suffering animals, the image supplied is of a female being who desires consummation through consumption. A consumption through which she will literally disappear. In making misery sexy, misogyny is swallowed along with every bite of meat or dairy or egg. As sex roles bend to gender diversity and gender equality, eating fewer animal products helps us all divest from the sexual politics of meat. Maybe tofu sausages are as destabilizing of the norm as that beer ad suggested!

THE INNER LIVES OF FARMED ANIMALS

■ Jacy Reese

Researcher at Animal Charity Evaluators and community organizer in the effective altruism movement

■ Peter Singer

Ira W. DeCamp Professor of Bioethics at Princeton Uni-
versity and author of over forty books, including *Animal
Liberation*, *Practical Ethics*, *The Life You Can Save*, and *The
Most Good You Can Do*

Caretakers and visitors know Nikki as the loud, social mother pig who's always been incredibly protective of her piglets. Since Nikki came to Farm Sanctuary in 2008, the caretakers have gained her trust, and she has become comfortable letting them take care of her children.

These social behaviors—protecting loved ones and building relationships with newcomers—are shared through much of the animal kingdom. But we can ask more about what a pig can do, to inform our decisions on how to treat them.

For example, Cambridge neuroscientist Dr. Donald Broom commented that pigs are more intelligent than human three-year-olds. In one cognitive test, Dr. Broom found that pigs could use a mirror to find food hidden behind a wall, a cognitive feat many would guess is limited to humans and other primates.

But are the intelligence and perceptive capabilities of pigs shared by other creatures we eat for food, such as chickens and fish?

Chickens: Biologist Dr. Carolynn Smith and science writer Sarah Zielinski remarked in a 2014 *Scientific American* article that "Mounting evidence indicates that the common chicken is much smarter than it has been given credit for." In one experiment, chickens showed the ability to delay gratification (something many adult humans still struggle with) by choosing a six-second wait for more food instead of a two-second wait for less food.

Fish: Fish biologist Dr. Culum Brown remarks that there is a "large gap between people's perception of fish intelligence and the scientific reality" and that "fish perception and cognitive abilities often match or exceed other vertebrates." Their many cognitive talents include tool use, such as hitting a shellfish against a rock to break it open.

But we must also ask whether this intelligence is even necessary for our moral consideration. We certainly don't think more intelligent humans matter more than less intelligent ones, so why would we apply this standard to nonhuman animals? As Jeremy Bentham succinctly phrased it, "The question is not, Can they reason? nor, Can they talk? but, Can they suffer?"

This question has an even clearer answer than that of animal intelligence. A group of prominent scientists—including neuroscientists Jaak Panksepp and Christof Koch—gathered in 2012 to assert the consciousness of nonhuman animals. This scientific fact raises important questions for the callous way we treat farmed animals.

In the summer of 2008, months of heavy rain led to severe flooding in the Midwest United States. Pig farmers in this area abandoned their facilities, leaving behind countless animals without any defense from the rising waters. Many of these animals drowned. A few survived the initial flooding, only to be stranded without food or water.

A team of animal activists, including caretakers from Farm Sanctuary, traveled to Iowa to help some of these pigs. Among the survivors was Nikki, the protective mother, and the piglets she birthed while stranded on a levee.

If she were left on the farm and the floods hadn't come, she would have continued living as most mother pigs do—in a tiny metal enclosure so small she couldn't even turn around. As the Humane Society of the United States puts it:

> They chew on the bars, wave their heads incessantly back and forth, or lie on the pavement in an apparent state of dejection. Nearly immobilized, the pigs spend months staring ahead, waiting to be fed, likely going out of their minds.

If Nikki were born an egg-laying hen, she would be in no better situation. She would probably live in a similarly cramped space, called a battery cage, which is so small that she wouldn't even be able to spread her wings. She would suffer constantly from poor health and stress due to the confinement and inhibition of natural behaviors like nesting and dust-bathing.

If Nikki were born a chicken raised for meat, instead of a small cage she would live in a crowded, dirty shed with thousands of other birds. She would grow at an unnaturally fast rate, leading to chronic pain. Her legs might not be able to hold the weight of her massively overgrown breasts, and she would spend most of her life crippled and sitting in her own feces.

These are only a few of the shocking details that are standard practice in animal agriculture. An estimated 99 percent of farmed animals in the United States are raised in "factory farms" where extreme confinement and the other worst forms of abuse are commonplace.

It's tempting to conclude that we can resolve these issues simply by supporting farms that raise animals with happy lives, either through government regulation or consumer pressure.

Unfortunately, neither of these options seems promising as a long-term solution. The resources needed to enforce such extensive regulations make it unrealistic to expect that they could be implemented across every farm, unless the size of the animal agriculture industry is drastically reduced. And from a consumer perspective, it's incredibly difficult to actually monitor all our consumption, including restaurant visits and everything else, sufficiently to have any reasonable confidence in the welfare of each animal involved. Even if we could track specific farms, it would be challenging to see beyond what farmers and food companies present to the public, which is often very different from the harsh reality the animals endure.

Many people are beginning to combine this understanding of our horrific food system with the recognition that farmed animals are sentient individuals, much like our dogs and cats at home. They are reaching the conclusion that animal agriculture is nothing less than a moral disaster. Historian Dr. Yuval Noah Harari has called it "the worst crime in history."

One way to address this pressing issue is through our consumption of animal products. Reduce now, and next month, reduce more. Maybe you'll get to zero, and anyway, you'll be doing less harm.

BUDDHISM AND BUTCHERY

David Barash

Evolutionary biologist, professor of psychology at the University of Washington, and author of *Buddhist Biology: Ancient Eastern Wisdom Meets Modern Western Science*

Buddhists are often assumed to be unworldly, wrapped up in their own personal enlightenment, sitting cross-legged in deep meditation and thus indifferent to the "outside" world. Although in some extreme cases this may be true, the reality is that engaged Buddhism has a lengthy and noble history, beginning when the Buddha is said to have gone out into the world for the benefit of "all sentient beings."

There are many reasons for everyone—even non-Buddhists—to reduce their consumption of meat. But those wanting to add a potent philosophical reason for doing so, especially one that is remarkably consistent with modern science, would do well to consult the astoundingly modern wisdom of an ancient Eastern tradition.

Among the key precepts of Buddhism is the concept of interdependence—pratitya-samutpada—the message that there is no "inside" as distinct from the "outside." (What did the Buddha say to the hot dog vendor? "Make me one with everything.") It is the eighth-century Indian scholar and philosopher Santideva who left us perhaps the earliest clear statement deriving ethical precepts from Buddhist teaching. "Just as the body, which has many parts owing to its division into arms and so forth, should be protected as a whole," he wrote, "so should this entire world be protected, for it is differentiated and yet it has the nature of the same suffering and happiness." David McMahan points out that similar statements can be found in East Asian texts, such as the writing of Korean monk Gihwa, from the early fifteenth century: "Humaneness implies the interpenetration of heaven and earth and the myriad things into a single body, wherein there is no gap whatsoever. If you deeply embody this principle, then there cannot be a justification for inflicting harm on even the most insignificant of creatures."

Arguably one of the first Buddhist precepts is ahimsa, or non-harming, a notion that has long been interpreted to refer to living things generally, not just to other people. The English word *compassion*, crucial to Buddhist practice, is significant in its derivation as well as its meaning. It originates in the word *passion*, which refers not to erotic desire but to "suffering," as in the Christian usage— the "passion of Christ." Compassion therefore bespeaks "suffering with" and is intimately related to "awareness of being connected."

Suffering with, however, has not always translated into identifying with, especially among people reluctant to acknowledge their connectedness with the animal world. "In an aversion to animals," wrote the early-twentieth-century philosopher and cultural critic Walter Benjamin, "the predominant feeling is fear of being recognized by them through contact. The horror that stirs deep in man is an obscure awareness that in him something lives so akin to the animal that it might be recognized." In effect, then, the widespread fear of being connected to animals is due in large part to an often-unacknowledged awareness that there may be a connection between man and beast.

Although Buddhism is unquestionably more biofriendly than the Abrahamic Big Three (Judaism, Christianity, and Islam), it was never nature worship, especially not in its earlier, formative stage. Thus traditional Buddhist teaching identifies a hierarchy in nature, with animals located below humans, although connected to them. At one point, the renowned fifth-century Buddhist commentator and sage Buddhaghosa noted that there is more "demerit" in killing a large animal than a small one. In other words, killing an elephant generates a greater karmic burden than killing a mouse, which in turn is more burdensome than killing a fly. This isn't so much because the

elephant is especially valued relative to the mouse, but rather because it takes more energy—and thus intention—to kill a larger animal. In addition, monastic Buddhist law holds that killing a human
is a far greater offense than is killing an animal, even though traditional Buddhists also maintain that any creature could have been
one's great-great-grandmother. (I wouldn't eat any of my immediate
ancestors, although I do sometimes eat meat.)

No human society is without admiring references to animals. We
are told to soar like an eagle, be as strong as a bull, busy as a bee, and
so forth. But it is one thing to be like an animal and quite another to
face the idea that humans and animals are deeply and irrevocably
united via our anatomy, physiology, behavioral inclinations, and lit-
eral evolutionary heritage. The modern Zen master Thich Nhat Hanh
goes beyond the teaching of earlier Buddhists and urges us to face
those facts of intimate connectedness, reminding us that having
done so, we are compelled to behave differently as a consequence.
Important words for everyone, but especially for those committing
to a life with less meat:

> "A human being is an animal, a part of nature. But we single our-
> selves out from the rest of nature. We classify other animals and
> living beings as nature, acting as if we ourselves are not part of it.
> Then we pose the question, 'How should we deal with Nature?' We
> should deal with nature the way we should deal with ourselves! We
> should not harm ourselves; we should not harm nature. . . . Human
> beings and nature are inseparable. Therefore, by not caring prop-
> erly for any one of these, we harm them all."

DEVIANT EATS: LEARNING FROM MISFITS

▌ Alexa Clay

Co-author of *The Misfit Economy: Lessons in Creativity from Pirates, Hackers, Gangsters, and Other Informal Entrepreneurs*

What do moonshine, camel milk, and guayusa tea leaves all have in common? They were all goods that once belonged to the informal, "gray market" economy. In Appalachia, moonshine or "hooch" was made by poor farmers who could turn their corn crop into alcohol and earn extra money without paying taxes. Moonshine eventually became its own currency, tradeable in some towns in east Tennessee for other goods and services. The origin of NASCAR racing is also tied to moonshine; old bootleggers delivering backwoods liquor from the southern Appalachians were forced to learn racing techniques to outrun the police.

I've been thinking a lot about these sorts of shadow economies lately, each populated by its own cohort of underground innovators. As part of my research, I've traveled around the world, speaking with misfits in India, Brazil, Kenya, and China and across rural and urban America. The question I've been asking is simple: What can we learn from the leaders of gray market and informal economies that we can apply to the mainstream economy? An iteration of that question is one I'd love to explore here: How can hackers, moonshiners, Luddites, gangsters, and other outlaws help us alter our own food consumption?

This isn't a trendy VICE article about "eating like a gangster" or tips for "losing weight on a prison diet" (although apparently in Japan there are now prison-themed restaurants). Rather, I have come to believe that people who regularly try to stay one step ahead of the system might have something surprisingly profound to offer those of us looking to develop our own insurgent eating habits. Here are a few concrete tips from misfits.

EAT LIKE A LUDDITE

Camel milk, once illegally sold by Amish farmers through informal buyer's clubs, can now be found at specialty retailers across the United States. While we don't often turn to Luddites—by which I mean, those who have resisted modern technology—when we think about innovation, communities like the Amish might have a lot to teach us about creative and quirky local food production. Although they do eat meat, the Amish aren't gluttons, and they attempt to use as much of the animal as possible. Many Amish, for example, eat scrapple, a dish made from leftover animal trimmings mixed with cornmeal or flour and served at breakfast time. Compared to many urbanites, the Amish also eat less store-bought food, which means they have more control over where their food was originally sourced. Around the United States, there are now buyer's clubs for local produce and seasonal groceries that you can have delivered directly to your door, while still supporting nearby farmers.

CREATIVELY REUSE LEFTOVERS

Moonshiners were famous for making a profit from their leftovers. Even today, the mash left behind by moonshine production can be used as food stock for pigs and cows. This does involve slight animal drunkenness, however, so best not to try it at home (see YouTube videos as evidence). That said, the concept of "zero waste" production is widespread within the informal economy. Waste pickers in slums around the world exhaustively go through trash heaps to recover items for reuse. The spirit of frugality and resourcefulness is one that used to underscore much of our food consumption but seems to have been lost in an age of mass food production. Today, over $1 billion a year is spent disposing of Americans' food waste. We need to bring back the spirit of creative reuse. In Berlin, London, and New York, I've taken part in food waste dinner parties, where friends get together and bring leftovers from their homes—food they won't use—and test their collective cooking skills by turning these scraps into an exquisite culinary experience. It's been incredible to see what leftover macaroni, beets, and orphan vegetables can do in the hands of creative chefs.

EMPLOY RITUALS

In Amazonian villages in Ecuador, Guayusa leaves are made into a tea that is part of a spiritual practice of the community. Villagers get together, share ancestral stories, and drink the homebrew. In modern life, many of our eating and drinking practices have become devoid of meaning or ritual. The tyranny of time poverty means that we can't appreciate the things we put in our bodies. Bringing ritual back into food consumption is also a way to eat with more intentionality and awareness. In accordance with our Greek heritage, every Easter my family comes together to roast a lamb on a spit. It's a ritual. For me, meat consumption is part of the way I connect with people. Similarly, when I travel and stay with families in remote parts of the world, I am often served meat. Refusing the food feels ungrateful and would further cement my outsider status. But accepting the food creates a feeling of familiarity and intimacy, just as it does with my own family. Limiting my meat consumption to these sorts of ceremonial or ritualistic instances has made meat consumption part of a sacred occurrence, rather than a default lifestyle.

Ultimately, if we are to take any advice from hackers about our food system, it should be "don't take on the whole system at once." Part of why reducetarianism appeals to me is that it's not asking us to drastically rethink our entire food system. Instead, we are encouraged to focus on the small and measured hacks we can make in our own lives that in turn may help inspire a different way of thinking about meat eating. If drug kingpin and cocaine trafficker "Freeway" Rick Ross can survive as a vegan in prison, I'm pretty sure we can all find a few ways to bring intentionality into our own diets.

FROM MRES TO McRIBS: MILITARY INFLUENCE ON AMERICAN MEAT EATING

▌ Anastacia Marx de Salcedo

Author of *Combat-Ready Kitchen: How the U.S. Military Shaped the Way You Eat*

It's three in the morning, still hot, barely any traffic on the six-lane highway that runs from Kuwait City to Iraq. High above the LSA (logistics support area) in a wooden tower, the soldier on guard duty rips open an MRE (meal, ready to eat), more from boredom than from hunger. He gropes around inside the thermoplastic wrapper and pulls out a flat brown box—the entree and a flameless heater. He pours in water from his hydration bladder, activating a heat-generating chemical reaction. In two minutes, he's tucking into warm beef brisket with a plastic spoon. Mmm.

Just like mom's.

Except the sauce-coated meat has been assembled from various pieces of tissue from a mechanically harvested carcass, mixed with numerous familiar and unfamiliar ingredients, packaged half a world away, and stored for years. Of course, it's a combat ration, so you'd expect sustenance made for these special and extreme circumstances—guiding down a helicopter, inspecting civilian vehicles at a checkpoint, digging a foxhole—might be different from civilian fare.

But in this you'd be wrong.

For a century, the U.S. military has been deeply involved in food science and the American food system, leading the shift from from-scratch meals consisting of local ingredients to prepared and convenience foods put together by distant producers and manufacturers. Nowhere is that influence more apparent than in meat.

Until the twentieth century, having a bone in our dinner had been an insurance policy—an indispensable feature for quick and easy identification of the animal and body part in question, as well as a vital clue as to its overall fitness for consumption. Only the poor gnawed on unrecognizable remnants, mostly in stews and soups.

Then came World War I. The military and its meatpacking friends in Chicago suddenly found they needed to supply 4.7 million troops with a pound of protein a day. Obviously it couldn't send whole carcasses overseas—not in such large quantities. Desperate to keep supplies running, the U.S. Army Quartermaster Corps worked with Hormel & Company to cut meat off the bone, pack it in boxes, and freeze it for transport in refrigerated holds. The results caused army bigwigs to do a little jig: A quarter carcass weighed 25 percent less without its bones, fat, and cartilage. When frozen into a rectangular solid, wrapped in burlap and waxed paper, and stacked, it occupied 60 percent less space on crowded trains and ships. On the downside, army cooks were none too happy about having to hack apart the contents with an ax, and recruits grumbled about the unappetizing brown color left by slow freezing. Nonetheless, by World War II, the Chicago meatpacking companies Armour and Swift had gotten in on the act, working with the Navy Veterinary Corps to invent new, more efficient deboning techniques, sort the meat by class, and flash freeze the flesh so it maintained a fresh appearance and texture.

Crowed the Defense Department in 1946, "Military advances in beef processing have made the beef ration a reality almost everywhere our present global Army may be. The Army has put boneless beef—frozen fresh and packed . . . on a basis where further experimentation is not necessary. It is now ready for civilian use."

Not quite.

In fact, it took the rise of the supermarket and the replacement of the old meatpacking business model (traditional butchery by tradesmen in cities along train lines) with a new one (assembly-line butchery by unskilled workers near rural feedlots along the federal highway system)—before civilians accepted the economic and practical benefits of boxed, boneless meat. Between 1963 and 2002, the percentage of boxed beef shipped from the nation's largest slaughterhouses increased from less than 10 percent to 60 percent of total sales, and now accounts for more than 90 percent of the beef sold in supermarkets.

The military, however, didn't stop with deboning. As soon as boxed meat was widely available, army brass set itself the modest goal of reducing the meat bill by 60 percent. It would buy the cheapest parts, and figure out a way to make them look and taste like the more desirable whole-muscle cuts.

Army food scientists went into the laboratory and began to fiddle, as well as to contract universities and the industry for outside research. They and their collaborators improved meat-flaking equipment; invented meat glue (a mixture of meat ooze, salt, and other chemicals); and discovered that adding phosphate improved juiciness, texture, and flavor. Together, these developments allowed them to paste together bits and scraps that could then be molded into a chop, cutlet, or steak tasting roughly like the real thing. By 1972 the army's fake-muscle-cuts project had successfully manufactured pilot runs of grill steaks, Swiss steaks, minute steaks, and breakfast steaks. It started serving the troops restructured veal cutlets in 1976, followed by lamb and pork chops and, somewhat later, beefsteaks. Soon, these Franken-foods were standard fare in the MRE.

Five years later, lured by the prospect of making something from almost nothing, restructured meat began to appear on fast-food menus. Working with army contractors, McDonald's began to serve delicacies such as the McRib, an ersatz baby back rib. (The item was so disdained by customers the first year that the monster restaurateur had to give it away to get people to try it.) Other chains soon followed suit, as did the consumer meat-processing industry. University and industry food-science departments looked for ways to further reduce manufacturing costs—this included hot deboning (while the corpse is still steaming), desinewing, mechanical separation (pushing a carcass through a sieve), blending fat and trim into protein "sludge," and collection of plasma for use as a plumper.

Consumption of restructured meat products exploded during the 1990s and early years of the 2000s—so much so that in 1997 the Census Bureau had to add a new industry code, nonpoultry meat processing, which that year generated $24 billion in sales. By 2007, it accounted for $37 billion.

Americans began the twentieth century clinging to their T-bones and prime ribs. But, thanks to the military, we no longer demand bodily evidence as to the origins and wholesomeness of our dinner—nor do we care if our entrée was made from the unappealing leftovers from butchering an entire herd or flock. In fact, we now prefer eating animals in the forms pioneered by the army: boneless and restructured. Bon appétit, America.

GOING "COLD TOFU"

■ Marc Bekoff

Author of *Why Dogs Hump and Bees Get Depressed* and *Rewilding Our Hearts: Building Pathways of Compassion and Coexistence*

While it would be best for the animals—and the planet—if everyone could eliminate consumption of animal products immediately, some people may have an easier time adjusting their diet more gradually. I like to call this approach, going "cold tofu." Clearly, there are many arguments for why it's not ethical to kill animals for food. Each of us can make a positive difference in the quality of ecosystems, our own health, and the lives of billions of other animals by changing our meal plans.

A good place to start is with meat produced on factory farms. This type of mass-produced food is the source of untold pain, suffering, and death. Really, they shouldn't be called farms at all—they are heartless, hellish factories in which billions upon billions of animals die terrible deaths due to greed and laziness. If you eat, for example, five cheeseburgers over the course of seven days, make a pact with yourself to slowly replace a few patties each week with a vegetarian or vegan alternative. A slow transition is better than no transition, and it could actually result in more permanent changes depending on your habits.

As I point out in my book *The Animal Manifesto*, we all need to

ask, "Who's for dinner?" not "What's for dinner?" when we're making decisions about our meals. The word *who* makes it clear that the
billions of food animals killed to feed us are in fact sentient beings.
I have found that merely thinking of who might be winding up in
your mouth is a helpful reducetarian strategy. There is no doubt
that animals suffer and cry out for help when they're being prepared for meals. The entire process is built on a foundation of cruelty, from the way these animals are raised, to their transportation
to the torture chambers of factory farms, to the final days and
hours of their lives as they await their turn surrounded by the
sights, sounds and smells of slaughter. Not to mention the fact that
when the "death blow" eventually comes, it is often delivered inefficiently, prolonging the experience and not instantaneously ren-
dering the animal unconscious as existing laws require. The last
paragraph of James McWilliams's 2015 book *The Modern Savage*
says it well:

> What I'm asking you to imagine is thus a movement that requires
> us to become more emotionally in tune with animals, ethically con-
> sistent in our behavior, and better informed about the evolution-
> ary heritage we share with sentient creatures. This movement,
> whether we join it all at once or gradually, with immediate zeal or
> reluctantly, will, in the end, triumph over industrial agriculture be-
> cause it will be, above all else, a bloodless revolution based on com-
> passion for animals, the environment, and ultimately ourselves.

Science clearly shows that factory farming is not sustainable. It
is an utter waste of water, land, other resources, and of course, the
lives of billions of animals. The award-winning documentary *Cow-
spiracy* is another great source for information on this topic. Some
would like to see the world become vegan. In my opinion this is a
wonderful goal, albeit an unrealistic one. But this doesn't mean we
can't make significant inroads toward reducing ecological devasta-
tion, food-related diseases, and animal suffering. And it's simple to
do. We're all responsible for the decisions we make about what—or
more accurately who—winds up in our mouths. Slowly but surely
transitioning into a meat-reduced society is a good place to start.

CHRISTIANITY'S COMPLICATED RELATIONSHIP TO FOOD

◼ Karen Swallow Prior

Author of *Booked: Literature in the Soul of Me* and *Fierce Convictions: The Extraordinary Life of Hannah More—Poet, Reformer, Abolitionist*

Some of the first words spoken to humankind in the biblical story of creation are about eating. One of the Christian church's defining rituals—communion—is a meal. In many Christian denominations, especially my own Baptist tradition, celebrations and lamentations alike center around the potluck supper. And the final vision for believers given in the Book of Revelation is a wedding feast.

Within this broader connection to food, however, Christianity's relationship with meat is even more complex. The Bible is clear that before the fall, Adam and Eve did not eat meat. In the beginning, no meat was eaten. As God tells Adam and Eve in Genesis:

> I give you every seed-bearing plant on the face of the whole earth and every tree that has fruit with seed in it. They will be yours for food. And to all the beasts of the earth and all the birds in the sky and all the creatures that move along the ground—everything that has the breath of life in it—I give every green plant for food.

It wasn't until after the great flood that God allowed the eating of meat. "Everything that lives and moves will be food for you," God continues in Genesis. "Just as I gave you the green plants, I now give you everything." Even so, many Old Testament laws restricted what meat could be eaten and how it was to be prepared—for many observant Jews, these laws help determine what food is considered kosher.

Further complicating Christian views toward eating meat are passages in the New Testament that essentially overruled older dietary constraints. Thus many different approaches to eating meat are found among Christians today, from the vegetarian lifestyle to the nonbinding standards of the Old Testament to the New Testament's open-ended approach. As I said, it's complicated.

Besides the biblical ambiguity, contemporary American Christianity remains heavily influenced by consumer culture. Most of the U.S. population, Christians included, rely on cheap, easy, and mass-produced food. We tend not to question the means of production any more than we do the other products we buy. In this cultural context, the reducetarian approach is especially helpful in upholding Christian principles

First, moderation is a tenet highlighted throughout the Bible. A verse in the Book of Philippians exhorts Christians to be known for their moderation. The Book of Proverbs is filled with admonitions to live in moderation; this one specifically addresses the eating of meat: "Be not among drunkards or among gluttonous eaters of meat." Self-control in general is considered one of the defining characteristics of the believer.

Reducetarianism also supports the Christian belief that the body is the temple of the Holy Spirit, an ideal that emphasizes bodily health and integrity. Some Christians interpret this tenet more strictly than others, adopting positions against smoking, drinking alcohol, and getting tattoos. But all Christians should be concerned about the food they eat. In his book, *What Would Jesus Eat?*, Don Colbert, MD, explains that in the Bible, gluttony "is not simply eating large quantities of food" but "also involves eating the wrong kinds of food." Many current health guidelines suggest Americans already include too much meat in their diets. Colbert argues that "God's initial plan" was for humans to be vegetarians, as evidenced by the long lives of many of the characters in the Old Testament, the period before God permitted eating meat. He explains that while humans are omnivores, "capable of living on both plant and animal foods," our bodies are actually "better suited for consuming more plant than animal products."

God gave many instructions, recorded in the Old Testament and later expanded in the Jewish Talmud, concerning the proper way to slaughter and prepare meat. With the benefit of modern science, we can see now that these ancient laws may have been designed in part to promote both human health and the humane treatment of animals used for food. The methods generally emphasized killing animals with the least amount of suffering possible. This is important for both animal and consumer because research shows scared food animals release a flood of potentially harmful hormones into their bodies during the slaughtering process.

Then there is the Christian mandate to be good stewards of God's creation. Few today associate animal welfare with Christianity, yet both the Bible and the ancient Christian church are full of stories promoting the protection of all creatures, big and small. Ignoring the rather classic example of Noah and his Ark, verses throughout the Bible speak of humans' obligation toward animals. "The righteous care for the needs of their animals," exhorts one Proverb. Church history, meanwhile, is filled with examples of leaders who spent a great deal of their lives caring for animals, from Basil of Caesarea to Saint Francis of Assisi and Thomas Aquinas.

And finally, there is the example of Jesus Christ himself. As Colbert explains in *What Would Jesus Eat?*, Jesus's diet would have been mostly plant-based, full of Mediterranean fare: lots of bread, lentils, olive oil, vegetables, dates, nuts and fish, and little red meat and poultry. Jesus, too, spoke out about the need to treat animals with compassion. Take this iconic passage in the Gospel of Matthew. "Are not two sparrows sold for a penny?" Jesus asked. "And not one of them will fall to the ground apart from your Father." It is not surprising that one of Jesus's nicknames is the Good Shepherd.

Clearly, Christian teachings on moderation, healthy bodies, and good stewardship embody reducetarian principles. It is my hope more Christians will consider eating less meat, from both a personal and a faith-based perspective.

TECHNICOLOR MEATSCAPES: WELCOME TO A POST-ANIMAL BIOECONOMY

▌Meera Zassenhaus

Assistant at New Harvest

Meat is composed of, in descending order: water, protein, fat, soluble organic material (amino acids, vitamins, carbohydrates), and minerals (most notably phosphorus and potassium). The recipe for beef differs, of course, from that for pork, just as a marbled steak is not the same as a lean one. And yet, these basic ingredients remain the same.

The art of cooking is figuring out how to manipulate these ingredients; how to undulate flavor through layers of texture and into the juice that dribbles down your chin. The actual making of the beef, chicken, or pork happens inside the cow, chicken, or pig, of course, each of whose DNA holds the ultimate recipe. Cooks can season, fry, or marinate, but even the most brilliant will always be constrained by the raw material at hand.

But suppose it were possible to expand the cook's jurisdiction to the making of the meat itself. So much of our energy is spent fumbling around as we crossbreed to figure out what combination of cut, aging, and feed will yield a perfectly marbled steak. What if, instead, we could play around—like a DJ on a soundboard—with the proteins and lipids and carbohydrates that dictate not just juiciness and tenderness but also the cells of the beef in question? Welcome to the post-animal bioeconomy.

Behold the carnery. It's a (as yet hypothetical) place where meat is made commercially, like in a brewery, via fermentation. Although it doesn't actually exist yet, the carnery is a thought experiment for a new paradigm of agriculture: cellular agriculture. Cellular agriculture is a way to harvest products like meat, milk, and eggs from cell cultures instead of actual livestock. It is an agriculture that deconstructs the burger to its most constitutive elements and then reconstructs it as a succulent patty, identical in every way except provenance. Winston Churchill actually predicted this revolutionized supply chain in December 1931, in an essay he wrote for *Strand* magazine. "Fifty years hence," he said, "we shall escape the absurdity of growing a whole chicken in order to eat the breast or wing by growing these parts separately under a suitable medium." Churchill was prescient, if overly optimistic (it's now thirty-four years past his prophesied "fifty years hence"). Not ones to be discouraged by a delayed timeline, however, a growing legion of biotechnology companies are pioneering an industry of animal-free animal products, in an effort to finally usher in just such a post-animal bioeconomy.

The process of culturing meat leverages existing technologies and techniques that are currently used in tissue engineering and regenerative medicine. To begin, we take a small sample of cells from an animal. The sample then proliferates in a nutrient-rich medium, inside a bioreactor. Cells are capable of multiplying so many times in a culture that, in theory, a single cell could be used to produce enough meat to feed the global population for a year. After they're done multiplying, the cells are attached to a sponge-like "scaffold" and soaked with nutrients. The resulting "cultured" meat is the same meat that would have resulted had those initial cells remained inside the animal—we simply used a bioreactor to take the place of an animal's body.

The field of cellular agriculture reimagines the way we produce and consume animal products. If meat is just a collection of muscle, fat, and connective tissues, then why raise an entire complex organism only to harvest these bits and pieces; why not start with the basic unit of life, the cell, to make the meat more efficiently? In fact, why stop at re-creating the shape, taste, and nutritional profile of existing meats? Let's create something new! To quote Julia Child, "Once you have mastered a technique, you hardly need to look at a recipe again and can take off on your own."

There is precedent for this kind of paroxysm of possibility. With the advent of cellular agriculture, cultured meat joins the ranks of cheese, yogurt, bread, beer, and wine—venerable mainstays of the modern diet and some of the earliest applications of biotechnology.

It was only after culturing milk, after all, that humans discovered kefir, yogurt, sour cream, and over 2,000 types of cheese. What might we discover as we culture meat? The gastronomic possibilities are practically limitless. But as the eighteenth-century epicure Jean Anthelme Brillat-Savarin once said, "The discovery of a new dish does more for human happiness than the discovery of a new star."

Cellular agriculture isn't just about meat, however. Already, people are working on making eggs without chickens, milk without cows, rhino horns without rhinos, and shark fins without sharks. Cellular agriculture suggests a way to emancipate the animal from the commodity supply chain.

Most of the controversy surrounding meat right now is based on the assumption that meat comes from an animal. As we become increasingly aware of the vulnerabilities in livestock supply chains as well as the very real and devastating impact animal agriculture is having on our health and the health of the planet, we are also being forced to think about how we can move toward a truly sustainable paradigm of food production. Strategies to reform the current system can do only so much. With problems of this magnitude, we need to be looking for an entirely new system.

Almost any paradox can be solved by abandoning a crucial assumption. If we abandon the assumption that an animal must be meat's bioreactor, our food can be disentangled from a bundle of uncomfortable truths and unsettling implications. Agriculture has always been a locus of innovation, and an early adopter of avant-garde technologies. Cellular agriculture is a natural evolution given the deeply ingrained culture of technological innovation. It sounds "revolutionary" and "disruptive," and it *is* revolutionary and disruptive. But it's also, frankly, just sensible.

EFFECTIVE REDUCETARIANISM

■ William MacAskill

Author of Doing Good Better: How Effective Altruism Can
Help You Make a Difference

The vast majority of the animals we eat are raised in factory farms. These are not humane places. The living conditions of factory farm animals have been extensively documented in books, magazines, and documentaries, so I will spare you the grim details here. The key issue is that they inflict severe and unnecessary suffering on animals merely for the sake of slightly cheaper produce. If you care about animal welfare—and most people do, as we see whenever someone mistreats a pet—then the conditions of animals in factory farms give you strong reasons to make some changes to reduce the amount of animal products in your diet.

However, this argument applies much more strongly for some animals than for others. This is because there is considerable variation in both the conditions animals are kept in and the number of animals needed to produce a given amount of calories. As a consequence, some types of animal produce involve a lot more animal suffering than others. Let us consider these two sources of variation in turn.

The first variation is in the animals' quality of life. Some farm animals live much worse lives than others. Of all the animals raised for food, broiler chickens, layer hens, and pigs are kept in the worst conditions, by a considerable margin. (In this discussion, I don't talk about fish, for two reasons. First, the data on both the number of fish used for human consumption and their quality of life are much more limited than the corresponding data for land animals. Second, there's more uncertainty about the sentience of fish relative to that of land animals than there is about the sentience of different land animals. Still, from the data that do exist, I suspect that cutting out fish is of comparable importance to cutting out chicken: the fish people eat have often been fed other fish, so the total number of fish deaths indirectly resulting from human consumption is very high, and it appears that the lives of factory-farmed fish are very bad too.) Bailey Norwood, an economist and agricultural expert, has estimated the welfare of different animals on a scale from –10 to +10, where negative numbers indicate that it would be better, from the animal's perspective, to be dead rather than alive.[1] Norwood rates beef cattle at 6 and dairy cows at 4. In contrast, his average rating for broiler chickens is 1, and for pigs and caged hens is 5. In other words, cows raised for food have lives that are comparatively good, in contrast with chickens, hens or pigs, who suffer terribly.

The second variation is in the number of animals needed to produce a given number of calories. A cow will feed an entire family for several months, whereas a chicken can be eaten in a single meal. In a year, the average American will consume the following: 28.5 broiler chickens, 0.8 layer hen, 0.8 turkey, 0.37 pig, 0.1 beef cow, and 0.007 dairy cow. One the basis of these numbers it would seem that cutting out chicken meat has a far bigger impact than any other dietary change.

Things are not quite so simple, however. Most broiler chickens live only for six weeks. Cows, by contrast, live for several years. Insofar as we care about how long the animal spends in unpleasant conditions on factory farms, it's more appropriate to think about *animal years* rather than about *animal lives*. If we adjust the figures in the previous paragraph so that they account for the varying lifespans of the different animal species in factory farms, the number of animal years that go into the average American's diet are as follows: 3.3 from broiler chickens (28.5 chickens consumed, each of which lives six weeks), 1 from layer hens, 0.3 from turkeys, 0.2 from pigs, 0.1 from beef cows, and 0.03 from dairy cows.

Combining these two considerations, we arrive at the following conclusion: *if you are only reducing the amount of animal products you consume, rather than going entirely vegetarian or vegan, the most effective way to reduce animal suffering is to stop eating chicken, then eggs, then pork.* Targeting the animal products that cause the most suffering ensures your efforts as a reducetarian have the highest payoffs in terms of animal cruelty avoided. If you are not prepared to go vegetarian or vegan, but you still want to reduce the negative impact that your diet has on animals, it is crucial that you focus on the worst offenders.

This shows the importance of *effective reducetarianism*, an example of a general approach I call *effective altruism*. Effective altruism is about asking, "How can I make the biggest difference I can?" and using evidence and careful reasoning to try to find an answer. It takes a scientific approach to doing good. Just as science consists of the honest and impartial attempt to work out what's true and a commitment to believe the truth whatever that turns out to be, effective altruism consists of the honest and impartial attempt to work out what's best for the world, and a commitment to do what's best, whatever that turns out to be.

As the phrase suggests, effective altruism has two parts. As I use the term, *altruism* simply means "improving the lives of others." Many people believe that altruism should denote sacrifice, but if you can do good while maintaining a comfortable life for yourself, that's a bonus, and I'm very happy to call that altruism. The second part is effectiveness, by which I mean doing the most good with whatever resources you have. It is important that effective altruism is not just about making a difference, or doing some amount of good. It's about trying to make the most difference you can. Determining whether something is effective means recognizing that some ways of doing good are better than others.

Reducetarians recognize that human diets vary *in degree* in the amount of suffering they cause, and on this basis seek to reduce the amount of animal products in their diet. *Effective* reducetarians accept this important insight, but combine it with the recognition that some animal products cause much more suffering than others. For effective reducetarians, the goal is not merely to eat fewer animal products, but to eat fewer of those products that cause the most suffering.

Ideally, I think we should eliminate as many animal products from our diet as possible. This is why I myself have been a vegetarian for many years. However, we must understand that many people are not prepared to go that far. Instead of blaming these people for failing to attain that ideal and implying that anything short of it is equally morally blameworthy, we should encourage them to be selective about the animal products they eat and to reduce those that harm animals the most.

YOU CAN DO ANYTHING!

▋ Myq Kaplan

Stand-up comedian

Eating less meat is good, do we agree? If yes, great! Are you eating less meat already? No? Go for it! Can't? It's hard? Maybe you're right. But I believe in you. You're a strong person. Undecided as to whether eating less meat is a good idea? Or would you like to be armed with witty (or non-witty) retorts that you can lovingly spew at people who disagree with you? Either way, the rest of this is for you.

What if I told you that you could live your life equally happily to how you live now, but with eating less meat? Would you believe me? Is it true? Probably. People always ask me how much I miss certain foods, but I honestly don't think about it that way. I eat a lot of food. Different kinds of food. And at every meal, there are certain things I'm *not* eating, but I'm not acutely aware of those lackings, because I *am* acutely aware of what is present. I'm grateful for what I have, much more than I am focusing on what I *don't* have. Some people don't even have food *at all*. I'm glad that I'm eating, period. If I'm eating something that tastes good (which I often am), then I'm happy about that. I'm not constantly wondering how it could be better. If you're only ever thinking about how things could be improved, maybe *that* is something that could be improved. Good luck!

And okay, yes, most of us were raised in a society where eating meat at almost every meal is the norm. Tradition! But if you go back through history, eventually you'll find that traditionally, meat wasn't involved in every meal, but rather it was a special occasion. In hunter-gatherer societies, gathering was a lot more reliable. Berries didn't run away. It was easier. And now, of course it *is* just as easy to go to the supermarket and gather meat, sure, but are you saying that laziness is what you value? Or just that you like to do what you're told, unquestioningly? Your parents ate meat, so you do. Past generations did it, so you do. Well, go back far enough and they didn't as much. So *now* what do you do?

Another thing that's not exactly traditional is the way that animals are treated in most of the places where people get their meat today. Whether you think we're the top of the food chain scientifically or if we were given dominion over the beasts of the field by a higher power, neither of those scenarios justify the unnecessary cruelty of factory farming conditions. God didn't tell Adam to name all of the creatures and then start cramming them up in sunlight-free rooms so they couldn't move and pump them full of hormones so they would produce the most tender results. Nor is that conclusion reasonable to come to from the fact that some of our teeth are sharp. So, eating less meat would help contribute less to that . . . and maybe that's not something you're actively concerned with, but would you consider at least being passively concerned about it? You're almost there, all you have to do is keep reading (not trying to hypnotize you, don't worry). If all other things were equal, and you could live basically the way you wanted no matter what, wouldn't you prefer there be less cruelty in the world? Just in general. Now, if you could alter your behavior in the slightest and then have a much larger effect, wouldn't you want to do that? You want to consider yourself a good person, right? Maybe you'll eat less meat, but you'll end up with more delicious, delicious feelings of superiority. Mmm, mmm.

Also, hey, are you trying to lose weight? Eat less meat! Less meat goes in, less weight goes on. Also you could go running more. Maybe you could run at people in the meat department of the supermarket and try to scare them away from it? You could read this to them if you want. You like scaring people, right? Why not! (Author's actual opinion: Fear is not my favorite.) What about the environment? Want more of it? Eat less meat! The more cows are kept in captivity, the more methane gas they're creating, and the closer the world gets to being just full of flatulence. You don't want that, do you? That would be weird if you did. I mean, it's fine to be weird. It's fine to want to live in a world of farts. But most people don't. You can help most people! And animals! And plants! And yourself! In so many ways! And all you have to do is eat less meat! I mean, not even zero. Zero's cool. But start with less! Think you can't do it? Well, I believe in you more than you do. You can too! You can believe in you more than you do. You can do the impossible! Or at least the illogical.

One last thing . . . if you're on board with all this (great!), but are concerned about the practical application, let me encourage you to not be concerned. The great thing about eating less meat is that it doesn't require you to think in absolutes, like "I will eat no meat." Maybe you want to eat no meat, but once in a while you slip up, then feel bad about slipping up, then drown your sorrow in a bucket of meat juice (I don't know what meat eaters do, really). But that's even worse! A negative feedback loop. A shame spiral. And it's not necessary. The world is not black and white. It's not all or nothing. If you make a rare mistake (by making a rare me-steak), you don't have to make more mistakes on top of it. You can accept and forgive yourself, acknowledge your limitations, and live both optimistically and practically. You can set realistic goals for yourself, like eating meat at one fewer meal a day, or one fewer day a week. You can do anything!

AN ANTHROPOLOGICAL SURVEY OF CARNIVORY AND MORALITY

▊ Avi Tuschman

Author of *Our Political Nature: The Evolutionary Origins of What Divides Us*

Human beings have adapted culturally—and even genetically, in the case of lactose tolerance—to thousands of highly specialized dietary niches. At the same time, eating a wide variety of plants and animals remains an ancient heritage; like numerous other mammals, we too are omnivores. Yet there's something peculiar about us: Even though the amount of animal protein in the human diet greatly surpasses that of other primates, our kind has felt far more conflicted than any other species over our carnivory. Simply put, there's tension between our humanity and our hunger. This paradoxical ambivalence is deeply rooted in our natural history and is reflected both in our religious traditions and in our political psychology.

Let's first review our evolutionary history in regard to meat consumption. Our closest living relatives are chimpanzees; our ancestors parted ways with theirs only 6 million years ago, according to DNA testing. Chimps live in relatively resource-poor environments, so they travel long distances in search of fruits, their staple food, and also to find seeds, resin, honey, and insects. In addition, chimpanzees are famous for forming hunting parties to kill red colobus monkeys and other medium-size game. Hunted meats, however, constitute only a very small proportion of the chimpanzee's diet. In fact, nonhuman primates in general subsist largely on fruits, leaves, and insects.

Our own ancestors likely evolved into modern humans while living in a woodland-savanna habitat similar to that of chimpanzees. Our ancestors' environment would have also provided sparse, high-value foods such as fruit and hunted meat. When we look at hunter-gatherer groups around the world today, however, the most notable thing about their diet is that they eat much greater amounts of hunted game than chimps do. Traditional foraging peoples put meat on the table with such frequency thanks to their advantage in intelligence over prey that can run, fly, or swim much faster than people. Even though chimps have much stronger arms and jaws than we do, humans have successfully hunted and eaten much greater amounts of animal protein due to our larger brains, and our enhanced capacities for communication, cooperation, and technology, including weapons and cooking. Vertebrate meat constitutes 30 to 80 percent of the diet of contemporary hunter-gatherer groups—more than ten times that of chimps.

Cooking with fire was a particularly important development in human evolution for two reasons: First, fire kills most pathogens and lowers the risk of eating meat. Second, cooking breaks down the connective tissue in meat and facilitates the digestion of this energy-rich food, reducing the work of our gut. Because our gastro-intestinal tract is as metabolically costly as our brain, there's a trade-off between the size of our guts and our brains, according to Leslie Aiello and Peter Wheeler's expensive-tissue hypothesis. Incorporating more cooked meat in our diet was therefore essential to evolving our notably small guts so we could afford to fuel our conspicuously large brains, which consume 20 percent of our body's energy.

The same powerful brain that has allowed humans to surpass other primates in meat consumption, however, also has much greater capacities for empathy and theory of mind. These faculties enable us to understand how similar we are to nonhuman animals. Just as we don't want to be killed and eaten, we know that neither does our lunch.

Herein lies the original conflict between our humanity and our carnivory: our close relatedness to meat. In his *On the Origin of Species*, Charles Darwin remarked "how infinitely complex and close-fitting are the mutual relations of all organic beings to each other." Since the nineteenth century, science has revealed that this interrelatedness is even greater than we could have imagined. The anatomy of a bat's wing is similar to the human arm not only because we share a distant common ancestor; we also share the same essential DNA blueprint with virtually every creature that has limbs. As evolutionary biologist Neil Shubin has emphasized, "We are not separate from the rest of the living world; we are part of it down to our bones and . . . even our genes."

Of course, we didn't need science to contemplate the deep connection between our humanity and our food. People have recognized this relationship for centuries—and we've also been denying it for just as long. After all, few thoughts can take one's appetite away as quickly. Both the recognition of this connection and its denial are reflected in our great religious traditions.

In the Judeo-Christian tradition, God says, "Let us make man in our image, in our likeness, and let them rule over the fish of the sea and the birds of the air, over the livestock, over all the earth, and over all the creatures that move along the ground" (Genesis 1:26). According to the Bible, then, humans are fundamentally different from animals, which are a divinely provided resource for our benefit and consumption. According to the Catholic Church, animals, unlike people, don't have souls that survive death—although Pope Francis recently unleashed a small scandal by suggesting that there's a place in heaven for pets.

In contrast with this Abrahamic doctrine that people have immortal souls while animals have only short-lived spirits, many Eastern religions hardly make as great a distinction. In Buddhism, neither humans nor animals have immutable or immortal souls. Both the Dalai Lama and Gautama Buddha are believed to have been animals in previous lives. Gautama's horse, Kanthaka, died of sadness when his owner left on his spiritual quest, but was reborn as a Brahmin and achieved enlightenment. Buddhism strongly emphasizes the mutual interconnectedness of life, and the ceaseless flow of energies between different life forms. No wonder, then, that vegetarianism is advocated in influential spheres of Indian religions like Hinduism and Buddhism—and is even mandatory in Jainism. By contrast, vegetarianism is not promoted by mainstream authorities in the Abrahamic faiths.

The beliefs and attitudes of coreligionists vary widely, of course, including in regard to eating meat. Different views toward carnivory are as common as liberal versus conservative opinions. As I've shown in my book *Our Political Nature*, human political orientation stems from three clusters of measurable personality traits that have substantial genetic and environmental components. This is true of religiosity, which is a facet of one of these clusters called tribalism. We can quantify religiosity according to participation in organized religious behavior, belief in life after death, and other measurements; when we do so, we find that higher levels of religiosity universally predict higher levels of political conservatism.

It's quite fascinating that the most culturally relative part of political orientation is religiosity. And there's no better example of this than these contrasting attitudes toward eating nonhuman animals: cultural conservatives in certain areas of Hinduism, Buddhism, and Jainism feel very differently toward meat consumption, on average, than culturally conservative Christians, Jews, or Muslims. And within each group, more liberal individuals are more likely to lean in the opposite direction on vegetarianism.

Whichever way one looks at it, eating meat tears at the conscience of our species. We've been conflicted between our hunger and our humanity. We've found ourselves pulled between our bodies and our intellect—between our instincts and our moral ideals. Every thinking person in today's globalized world must confront this ethical paradox, in addition to the numerous other environmental and health considerations that eating meat in today's industrialized societies entails. For these reasons, contemplated in depth in this book, reducetarianism is an excellent compromise.

THE POWER OF FILM TO EXPOSE THE MEAT INDUSTRY AND CHANGE LIVES

Mark Devries

Director of *Speciesism: The Movie*

Today's meat industry does everything it can to stop us from seeing and hearing what takes place inside factory farms. It has deployed tactics ranging from lobbying for the criminalization of hidden-camera investigations of agricultural facilities to paying for front groups to launch smear campaigns against the individuals and organizations that do such investigations. It does this, quite simply, because there is no more powerful indictment of the industry than a straightforward image of it.

I am a documentary filmmaker, and a primary focus of mine has been exposing the animal welfare and environmental impacts of factory farming. While directing my first documentary, *Speciesism:*

The Movie, I came face-to-face with one of the most disturbing and little-known environmental catastrophes in the United States. Thousands of factory pig farms dot the eastern North Carolina countryside, and within each one, hundreds or thousands of pigs spend their lives standing on concrete floors. Their waste falls through slats in these floors, and is collected in giant, open-air cesspools, often the size of several football fields, and often near homes and communities. Far more than cow manure, pig waste can produce a truly sickening odor while being flushed into the cesspools. As a result, neighbors' homes are regularly, and without any warning, invaded by the overwhelming stench of raw sewage. Most disturbingly, cesspools are emptied by having their contents sprayed high into the air, where the sewage turns into a fine mist that can settle on—and sometimes in—neighbors' homes.

I captured footage of these facilities from an airplane for *Speciesism: The Movie*, and returned to North Carolina recently to document them closer up using a camera-equipped drone. The resulting short documentary, at FactoryFarmDrones.com, far exceeded my expectations, now having been viewed over 18 million times between Facebook and YouTube. I believe that it was successful for the same reason that factory farms are hidden: When people can see what is taking place, they can see that something is wrong. Footage, whether collected undercover by employees or overhead by a drone, is one of the central keys to effecting change.

Film can also be used to solidify abstract ideas. When I began filming *Speciesism: The Movie* several years ago, I did not understand that I was documenting an unprecedented, historic, cultural shift in the way humankind views nonhuman animals. Now, things are changing at an even more rapid pace. In 2015 alone, a New York court discussed the prospect of viewing chimpanzees as legal persons; *The New York Times* ran a front-and-center opinion piece by a former animal experimenter denouncing his career's work; and Ringling Bros. announced that it would soon stop using elephants in its shows, to name just a few examples.

The argument for this change is straightforward: Among the most fundamental principles of all plausible ethical theories is that causing harm, all else being equal, is a bad thing. Nonhuman animals are capable of being harmed; in fact, the scientific evidence strongly indicates that they are capable of suffering physically and emotionally to the same level of intensity as human animals. Therefore, the unreflective assumption that nonhuman animals are ethically insignificant may reflect a form of prejudice, similar in kind to prejudices against groups of humans—speciesism.

My first thought upon hearing this argument was something like, this can't be right; there must be an obvious flaw, if I just think about it for a moment. So I thought about it, for more than a moment; then I read about it; then I interviewed some of the world's most influential scientists and scholars about it for *Speciesism: The Movie*. And the deeper I investigated, the more it seemed like— against everything I had been taught and grown up assuming about the status of humans in the world—there was indeed something to this philosophical argument, and it could not be ignored.

The first objection to taking nonhuman animals seriously would seem to be, "humans are in fact superior" (we're smarter, we use language, we create art . . .). The problem, animal advocates will quickly point out, is that many humans are not "superior" in any of these ways. There are young children, severely senile people, and intellectually disabled people who lack whatever special characteristic we might try to claim separates us and makes us more important. And yet, of course we do not consider these people to be outside our sphere of ethical concern. As a result, the characteristics they lack could not possibly be some kind of prerequisite for moral status.

The second inevitable objection is that even if we are not superior by virtue of some characteristic that we possess, is it not simply part of some natural order for us to consider other species less important? The problem with this argument is that, however one defines natural (perhaps "behavior that served a direct evolutionary benefit," or "behavior that existed before advanced technological civilization"), it will always include behaviors that are decidedly unethical. Racism, for example, appears to be a result of psychological tendencies that served direct evolutionary benefits, and warfare surely existed since long before advanced technology. Yet, the "natural-ness" of such behaviors hardly provides an argument against seeking to minimize and prevent them.

If we can no longer justify the traditional sharp ethical distinction between humans and nonhuman animals, it seems to follow that our view of humankind's place in the world must radically shift. We share this planet with countless other species, and our decisions—political and personal—affect them. One decision, though, stands out from the rest: Considering that billions of animals experience the most immense suffering conceivable in the factories where they are raised to become food, the present societal shift away from meat consumption may be among the most ethically significant events in our history.

THREE MENTAL HACKS TO HELP YOU BE A REDUCETARIAN

Nick Cooney

Author of *Change of Heart: What Psychology Can Teach Us About Spreading Social Change*

As you settle in to a cushioned, comfy booth at your favorite restaurant, your eyes slowly scanning the menu to see what you're in the mood for, it would seem that at this point your stomach is calling the shots. By and large we eat what we like, right?

Only, that's not really what's going on. Eating is in large part a psychological act. What we eat isn't just determined by our taste buds; it's also decided by our brains.

Consider for example how what we "like" tends to be foods heavy in ingredients that were hard to come by for our distant ancestors: fat, salt, and sugar. Right out of the gate, it's clear that what we think of as food preferences are really just you and me dutifully obeying our brain's commands to gravitate toward certain types of fare. And that's just scratching the surface. The fact is that our eating habits are driven in large part by the same psychological forces that drive all our other life choices.

One such force is what psychologists have dubbed the "status quo bias." We're hard-wired to think that the way things are right now is the way they should be. Another example is the power that social norms have over us. We care a heck of a lot about what other people are doing—either other people in general, or at least others in our social and peer groups—and we tend to copy them. A third and final example is what's called "loss aversion." We get very worried at the prospect of losing something we have, even if what we have isn't all that great.

What does all this mean when it comes to what's on our plate? It means that we don't eat a chicken sandwich just because we think it tastes good. We eat a chicken sandwich because we've eaten them before. We eat a chicken sandwich because we see other people eating them. And we eat a chicken sandwich because the idea of intentionally giving it up—of turning it down, even if we may want it—seems like a major sacrifice.

Which raises an important question: What do you do when, whether to boost your health, protect animals, or preserve the environment, you want to start eating fewer of those chicken sandwiches? What do you do when you want to start eating less meat in general?

If the idea of being a reducetarian interests you, but you're not sure you're ready to make the plunge and start cutting back on chicken, fish, and other meat, have no fear. It's just that old brain of yours, and those same psychological forces, trying to get in your way and hold you back from doing what you really want to do. The good news is, once you understand what your brain is up to, succeeding is just a matter of cutting back in a way that won't trip any of your mental alarm systems.

To that end, here are three mental hacks that will make eating less meat a breeze.

HACK ONE: GO WITH WHAT YOU KNOW

Like your taste buds, your brain is afraid of new things. Falafel, vegetarian sausages, tofu pad thai, meatless chicken nuggets, and quinoa are all delicious (and protein-packed) meat-free options. But if you've never had them before, the idea that skipping meat means having to venture into these uncharted culinary territories can be intimidating. "New and unfamiliar foods = bad and gross foods," your brain tells you.

Of course that's not true, and in time it would be great to occasionally try new dishes. But to start, just stick with meals you already know and love that happen to be meat free. Think pasta with marinara sauce, big hearty salads with lots of nuts, bean burritos packed with guacamole and salsa, and seasoned rice with stir-fried vegetables. Starting off with familiar meatless dishes will help you bypass your brain's constant fretting over anything new.

HACK TWO: MAKE FRIENDS

As much as we like to think of ourselves as strong, independent individuals, at heart we're all a bunch of copycats. If we're the only ones doing something, we get anxious. We don't want to stick out from the herd.

On the other hand, if we have just one or two other compatriots, we start to feel a lot more at ease. So when cutting back on meat, try to avoid going at it alone. Find a friend to do it with you, or if you have a romantic partner enlist him or her. Seek out co-workers or friends who are already reducetarians so you can ply them for meal tips and restaurant suggestions.

Tens of millions of Americans are cutting back on meat, so it shouldn't be too hard to find someone who fills the bill. But if you're having trouble, just go online. There are plenty of Facebook pages, community Meetup groups, and recipe Web sites where you can interact with people making the same healthy food choices as you.

HACK THREE: CROWD OUT MEAT

The idea that we might lose something we have is scary, whether that's a personal possession or the freedom to do something we like. The same is true with food. The idea of giving up a dish we enjoy, whether for one meal or forever, is not going to put a smile on our face.

So when going reducetarian, don't focus on giving up meat. Focus on piling your plate high with delicious meatless options until there isn't even much space left for it. Take a cue from some of the nation's foremost restaurateurs, who are turning meat from an entrée to a small side dish and letting vegetables, grains, and plant-based protein sources play the starring role.

Because you're not giving anything up, your brain won't worry about losing something it likes. And as you get used to plant-centered meals, your brain will soon latch on to those. In no time, you'll likely be telling yourself, "Give up my veggie chili? Never!"

Happy hacking, and happy meat-free eating!

TURNING TO TECHNOLOGY: MEAT AND ARTIFICIAL INTELLIGENCE

■ Stuart Armstrong

Author of *Smarter Than Us: The Rise of Machine Intelligence*

There is wisdom in accepting the inevitable, of making peace with that we cannot change and trying to transform only that which can be transformed. But those following this path must check, periodically, to make sure the inevitable has not suddenly become evitable due to the breathtaking speed and possibilities offered by ongoing technological innovation.

For many years, we assumed the torturous existence of billions of factory-bred farm animals was just such an inevitability. The blame for this particularly common problem is often placed at the feet of farming industrialists (the quaint concept of the "farmer" applies to an almost vanished entity), but such operators are merely working to satisfy a seemingly insatiable demand. Such producers are caught in a zero-sum race: Improving the lives of their animals requires costs that are difficult to pass on to the consumer without hurting their business. And yet, consumers are not particularly to blame either: paying for more expensive foods under some vague promise of "better treatment for the animals" feels both individually pointless and impossible to verify.

Legal remedies, too, are not particularly forthcoming. To legislate against the torture of food animals, lawmakers would need to be able to specify, in full and unambiguous text, exactly what constitutes acceptable quality-of-life standards for all food animals. This is an ethically and logistically difficult task. Indeed, there is a closely related problem in safe artificial intelligence (AI) research. For the purpose of instructing a potentially superintelligent AI to deal with us in a way we would want to be treated, we would need to specify what would constitute an acceptable life for a human being. At this point, there is an almost irresistible urge to moralize: "If we don't treat farm animals with compassion, why do we merit the same?" This urge needs to be resisted. It's very easy to ask people to behave better from a moral perspective, but such entreaties rarely work. Trying to create new, widespread cultural norms is probably the hardest and least successful way of accomplishing a goal.

Turning to technology offers much better options. As civilizations become richer and technology improves, issues that were previously believed to be facts of life become solvable problems. Worker safety laws, clean air and water acts, the removal of lead from gasoline, and the creation of natural reserves are all examples of what happens when the cost of doing the right thing becomes very low. Innovation affords us the luxury of making the world better.

For the food industry, innovations in cultured and plant-based meats are improving to the extent that we should no longer assume issues like animal cruelty are set in stone. Cultured meats are in their infancy, while plant-based meats are a more mature technology. But in both cases, they have nowhere to go but up. Animal-free meat products are going to become tastier, more nutritious, more marketable, and cheaper in the future. Someday soon, they may even eclipse the quality, taste, and price of factory-farmed products.

When this happens, we may start to hear a chorus of appeals to nature and tradition. It will be argued that factory farming produces jobs, maintains important rural traditions, or is simply more natural and healthier than its alternatives. Laws will likely be passed to defend our current farming industry, and politicians will speak in its defense. But the same irresistible market forces that protect factory farming today spell its future demise. Once the change is complete, we may even be able to admit that, yes, it was a hideous atrocity (people seldom admit aloud that reality constrains moral choices) and that the world is better without it. And then, the inevitable will have become, well, evitable.

BODY

Our bodies are our gardens—our wills are our gardeners.
—WILLIAM SHAKESPEARE

HOW MUCH MEAT ARE WE DESIGNED TO EAT?

■ Chris Stringer

Author of *Lone Survivors: How We Came to Be the Only Humans on Earth*

■ Brenna Hassett

Physical anthropologist at the Natural History Museum, London

Many people who are interested in eating a healthy diet have looked to the long trail of human history for an "ideal" diet. It is easy to see why we might want to look to the past, before some of the foods and lifestyle choices that seem so obviously dangerous to our well-being (like excess refined sugar or smoking) are things we associate with our modern age. However, there is a very important point to be made before we all run off and try to re-create the lives of our ancestors: Our species today is very different from that of our earliest ancestors, and we live in a world unimaginable to even our most recent ones. The choices we have about what to eat are very different from those of the earliest branches of our family tree.

Our species, modern *Homo sapiens*, is part of a long evolutionary lineage stretching, by definition, back to the beginning of life on Earth. No one is suggesting that we revert to the diet of the early single-celled organisms of several billion years ago and start trying to digest carbon dioxide. It's fairly obvious that our complex human bodies just aren't built for that sort of intake. However, once we get to the point in our evolution where our own zoological family, the Primates, evolved over 60 million years ago, it becomes very interesting to look at what our relatives and ancestors were doing and eating.

Between 4 and 7 million years ago there is a sparse fossil record in Central and East Africa which shows apelike creatures that nevertheless seemed to have walked upright more regularly than our closest living relatives, the African apes (gorillas and chimps). Their canine teeth were small and their molars had thick enamel, unlike those of African apes of today, suggesting they may have had a more humanlike diet. But like present-day apes they were probably largely vegetarian. This early phase of human evolution was followed by an australopithecine ("southern ape") phase of between 2 and 4 million years, and many species are known, especially in eastern and southern Africa. These early ancestors were adept walkers on the ground, but still climbed in the trees. Their diets seem to have varied from nuts, berries, and leaves in woodlands to sedges and grasses in more open country, but they probably at times ate insects and the meat of small game, as do modern chimps.

Between 2.5 and 3 million years ago, some members of this group began to increasingly process their food with stone tools and to eat larger quantities of meat, initially obtained through scavenging. The back teeth and jaws began to look more human as they reduced in size, and this marks the beginning of our genus *Homo* (humans). Early forms include the African species *Homo habilis*, from about 2 million years ago, and the widespread species *Homo erectus*, which survived into the last 500,000 years.

Our most recent human relatives occupied many different environmental niches. It is one of the hallmarks of our genus that *Homo* can be found for the last million years across much of the globe in savannas, woodlands, and alongside rivers and lakes with varied ecosystems. At least two other species have contributed their genetic material to our own, and we have good evidence for how one of them (*Homo neanderthalensis*) lived and dined. Hundreds of Neanderthal fossils have been found since the first was identified in 1856 in the Neander Valley, Germany, allowing us to build up a good picture of a typical Neanderthal body. They had big noses, large brains, and short, stocky physiques suited to living in cool environments. Neanderthals were skilled hunter-gatherers, built shelters, controlled fire, and buried their dead. They were certainly carnivores but they also ate other foods, although only limited evidence of the plants they consumed survives in the archaeological record. In Mediterranean regions they sometimes exploited marine resources such as shellfish and seals, but their use of aquatic foods was certainly more limited than that of modern humans. Evidence from regions like Gibraltar suggests that they also ate small game such as rabbits, tortoise, and pigeons.

Evolution has not been a straight and narrow path toward increased meat-eating in our lineage. We can see the same thing is true in other types of primates. What an animal eats might be based more on the environmental niche it occupies, and this reinforces associations between body shape and size and what an animal eats. Adorable, big-eyed tarsiers, about the size of a week-old kitten, require a very dense high-energy diet to survive—mostly at the expense of local insects and lizards. Gorillas on the other hand, are very large but spend most of their time eating very low-energy plant foods.

But if we want to understand what we as *Homo sapiens* are "supposed" to eat, we can take an even closer look at our own history. The archaeological record for our species is spread through all the points of the compass and across hundreds of thousands of years. We can find many different strands of evidence to build up a picture of what we used to eat from the artifacts left behind, looking at the shape of our bones and teeth, and even from analyzing the chemistry of ancient bones or food remnants in the tartar stuck on teeth. Evidence of what we ate can be as direct as finding a bin full of lentils in the 10,000-year-old houses of Çatalhöyük, Turkey, for example, or the burned and boiled bones of animals in trash pits at even earlier sites across the world.

So what do we know about what we are evolved to eat? From the teeth of people living even before the invention of farming, we see the proof of a fondness for carbohydrate-heavy plant foods, such as acorn, alongside a wide variety of other foods. Largely, what we see in the archaeological evidence is that for humans, pretty much anything would do (even, at times, the flesh of other humans). We can see that modern foragers, such as the Hadza of Tanzania, who have been pushed to the edges of habitable environments but who have also had a bit more time to hone their hunting skills than our ancestors, still get about 70 percent of their calories from plants.[1] For most of our history, humans have been keen on eating virtually anything, and the huge variety in our diets is a testament to our ability to survive when other species died out around us. There is no design that makes us need to eat a meat-heavy diet to be healthy. What we do have are a series of environmental, cultural, and social choices that humans, with our big brains and fancy tool-making abilities, can make about how and when (if at all) we consume meat.

LISTEN TO YOUR BODY

■ Elise Museles

Author of *Whole Food Energy: 200 All Natural Recipes to Help You Prepare, Refuel, and Recover*

Did you open this book hoping to find a magic formula for perfect health?

If you did, you are not alone. Many of us have spent years searching for a solution to better health and an easier relationship with food. I wish I could hand out a meal plan that would solve all of our problems!

In a perfect world, I'd give you a bullet-pointed list of foods that would give you boundless energy; maybe I'd share with you a group of foods you should avoid at all costs. In this fantasy world, I'd hand you a set of easy-to-follow rules that would help you feel your absolute best. All you would have to do is abide by that plan (or list or rules). In no time, you would look and feel amazing.

For better or for worse, there is no one-size-fits-all solution when it comes to health and nutrition.

This might feel a little disheartening. Many of us would love to put our health on autopilot. In fact, health can seem like a foreign land and most of us would appreciate a road map, written by someone who has been there. We'd love to find one type of exercise we like doing and then do it forever. We'd be happy with ten healthy, easy dishes and just cycle through those recipes, over and over and over. We'd want to figure out a specific diet, buy the appropriate cookbooks and tools, and then mentally check the box "got my health under control."

The truth is, no matter what any nutritionist, doctor, or specialist says, you are the only person who is truly an expert on your body. Sure, you can get nuggets of wisdom along the way, but no one else can tell you how your body feels after you eat an apple or a slice of bread or a handful of almonds . . . or even some buffalo chicken wings. No one else is looking through your eyes as they glaze over in a postdinner food coma. No one else experiences the energy coursing through your veins when you consume a bowl of quinoa and curried chickpeas.

Nutrition is highly individual, after all! While there are certainly guidelines and plans that are more right for you than others, you start feeling your best when you channel your inner nutritionist. Believe it or not, we all have one! When you can hear the voice inside, you find many of the answers you've been searching for all along. You will know which foods make you feel energized, uplifted, and nourished and which foods don't—even if they happen to be superfoods.

More than any single diet, you can get closer to finding health and balance when you learn to tune into your body. Even if I can't give you an airtight meal plan or a bullet-pointed list of must-eat foods, I can teach you how to listen to your body.

SLOW DOWN SO YOU CAN HEAR WHAT YOUR BODY IS TRYING TO TELL YOU

Many of us eat for the wrong reasons. We eat because we're bored or unhappy or because the clock says that it's dinnertime. We wait too long between meals, and then we're so hungry we eat anything that's available. When we eat too quickly, it's impossible to tune in to the signals that our bodies are sending us. How will you notice that you are not really hungry and food isn't the answer? How will you know whether your body can handle less animal protein at every meal if you're multitasking and rushing? How will you notice if you're satisfied when you eat your meals standing up, while reading your texts?

Give your body a chance to communicate with you. Regardless

of what you're eating, eat it sitting down. Chew and taste everything thoroughly. Bonus points for putting your fork down in between bites. Notice when you're full. When you give your body the chance to talk, you will be amazed by what it can tell you!

EXPERIMENT WITH NEW WAYS OF EATING AND LISTEN TO YOUR BODY WITH AN OPEN MIND

If you've spent your entire life believing that you need meat with every meal, you might imagine that reducing your animal protein consumption would result in low energy. But why not try it for two weeks? Check in with your body and observe with an open mind.

What happens if you add more fruits and vegetables? What happens if you consume less meat? Do you really feel better if you drink lemon water every morning? What if you ate something savory for breakfast instead of your usual fruit smoothie? What if you switched from animal-based protein to plant-based protein?

If you need a nudge in the right direction, here are five questions to ask yourself after you eat:

- How are my energy levels?
- Do I feel focused?
- How's my level of hunger—do I still feel full?
- What's my mood like?
- How are my cravings?

ADOPT AN ATTITUDE OF MORE

As you begin to reduce your meat intake and act as your own nutrition expert, you'll probably discover other foods that make you feel amazing and foods that . . . don't. Unfortunately, some of those foods that aren't the best choices for you might be delicious, all-time favorite recipes.

Rather than assuming a mind-set of restriction and denial, focus on what you can have by adopting an attitude of more—more color and more plants. Luckily for our health, more color and more plants happen to coincide with more nutrients and more whole foods!

Change your thought process from "I'm not allowed to eat barbecue chicken pizza" to "Gosh, these roasted vegetables are gorgeous." Move away from "What can I eat that's low in carbs if I'm not eating as much meat?" to "I can't wait to dish up a second helping of spaghetti squash!"

When we eat vibrant, colorful fresh food, we're removing the stress of dietary labels or theories. We free up our hearts and minds to focus on more important things. We're trusting ourselves enough to make delicious, healthful choices without crazy restrictions, and we're giving ourselves the gift of a lovely, thoughtfully prepared meal.

REMEMBER THAT WHAT'S RIGHT FOR YOU TODAY MIGHT NOT BE RIGHT FOR YOU TOMORROW

The food that works for today's long-distance run might not work next week when you're battling a cold. The meals that energized you while you were pregnant might make you feel slow and groggy when you're chasing toddlers.

You might be able to give up meat completely during the summer, but find yourself needing a bit more animal protein during the winter months. That's fine! Just stay in touch with your body, try new things, and see what works.

Ultimately, your body knows what's best. Release yourself from the expectations of what you "should" be eating and which foods "should" make you feel your best. Choose to view the foods in your pantry and refrigerator as a grand experiment.

Take a bite, open your mind, tune into your body, and see what happens!

YOU ARE WHAT YOUR MICROBES EAT

■ Alanna Collen

Author of *10% Human: How Your Body's Microbes Hold the Key to Health and Happiness*

In the West, we have access to the greatest variety of the most nutritious foods in the world, available all year round, despite the changing seasons. Yet every year, more people die worldwide of overnutrition and associated diet-related diseases than of undernutrition and starvation.

So-called diseases of civilization are on the rise: obesity and its attendant conditions—type 2 diabetes, heart disease, and liver disease; autoimmune diseases—from type 1 diabetes to lupus and celiac disease; allergies to everything from pollen to nuts; digestive disorders such as irritable bowel syndrome; and mental health conditions as ubiquitous as depression and as complex as autism. Although you'd be hard pressed to find anyone in the West who hasn't had experience of at least one of these conditions, they are relatively rare in the developing world, especially in areas as yet unsullied by the Western lifestyle, and, in particular, the Western diet that goes along with it.

Our diets are now so far removed from whatever is normal for humans, we're turning to communities in the developing world to learn how to eat, once again, for our health. Though life expectancy is shorter and child mortality higher in less developed countries, those who survive are far less susceptible to the kinds of illnesses that plague us in the West, largely as a result of our diets. So what is it that we're doing wrong, exactly?

The answer comes down to a misjudgment of our nutritional needs. Until recently, scientists addressing the surprisingly challenging question of "what should humans eat?" have focused their efforts on understanding exactly how we, first, digest, and, second, absorb the nutrients in our diets. Our small intestines are beautifully adapted for both these tasks. When we eat, this winding seven-meter-long tube is flooded with enzymes to break down our food into its component chemicals: proteins into amino acids, carbs into simple sugars, and fats into fatty acids and glycerols. These little molecules are small enough to be absorbed through the incredibly convoluted small intestinal lining—with its surface area equivalent to a tennis court—and into the bloodstream.

The remains of this digestive process—mostly indigestible plant parts we call dietary fiber—move on to the large intestine. Wider and shorter, with a surface area more akin to a double bed than a tennis court, this organ has been somewhat neglected in our explorations of the nutritional needs of humans. Its purpose seemed to be limited to fluid recovery and a little compacting of waste matter, but the emerging truth is that it provides a home to another organ. A forgotten, ignored organ that forms a connecting hub between our digestive, immune, and neurological systems, among others.

You see, only 10 percent of the cells that make up our bodies are human cells. The other 90 percent are microbes, mostly bacteria, and mostly living in our guts. Once seen as hangers-on, with little more to contribute to the running of the human body than a handful of vitamins and some unwanted gas, these 100 trillion individuals are more important for our health and happiness than we might ever have imagined. Through their intimate connection with our immune systems—the cells of which are also centered on the large intestine—our microbes influence our weight, our moods and behaviors, and our immune health. Dramatic rises in rates of allergies, autoimmune diseases, mental health conditions, and obesity are all tied to our treatment of our microbial allies.

So what's going wrong? There have been a few assaults on the microbiota, from frequent use of antibiotics, especially in childhood, to the decline in breast-feeding and the rise in caesarean section deliveries, many of which are medically unnecessary. But perhaps the biggest and most consistent change in our treatment of our microbes is the shift in our diets over time. As we struggle to work out what features of the modern diet are responsible for our poor health, scientists are studying the diets of those whose meals today still closely resemble those of their great-great-grandparents and beyond.

In one such study, scientists compared the diets of a group of city-dwelling Italian children with a second set of children living in a rural village in the West African country of Burkina Faso. In place of the typical Western diet of pizza, pasta, ice cream, and potato chips was a more traditional menu of grains, peas, and vegetables, supplemented with the occasional bit of chicken or even a handful of termites. It is not surprising that rates not just of obesity but also of allergies and autoimmune diseases are significant higher among European children.

You might guess where the Italian children are going wrong: their diet appears to be higher in fat. In fact, the composition of the diets of both groups of children was startlingly similar in terms of protein, fat, and carbohydrate content, although Italian children consumed more food in total. The biggest difference in macro-nutritional content was actually the amount of dietary fiber, with the African kids eating three and a half times more. The scientists' particular focus, though, was the impact of these differing diets on the children's microbiotas: the Burkinabe children's guts were dominated by fiber-loving species that were entirely absent from the guts of the Italian children and more often seen in the microbiotas of vegetarians in the West.

Though fiber is often said to have no nutritional value, this view ignores the huge impact it has on the diversity and makeup of the microbial communities in our guts. In turn, this impacts on our health. More precisely, it is not the species of bacteria we harbor that determine our health, but the compounds they produce, which we then absorb. In breaking down fiber, our microbes produce a new set of compounds, called short-chain fatty acids or SCFAs.

These molecules provide us with an invaluable set of services: They reduce inflammation by calming the immune system, which prevents allergies, autoimmunity, and even stops cancer cells developing. They feed the cells lining the gut wall, which reduces the risk of inflammatory bowel disease and bowel cancer. They keep the cells of the gut lining tightly bound together, preventing bacterial compounds from entering the bloodstream where they can affect how much energy we store as fat. And they even make us feel less hungry, telling the brain we have had enough. If fiber doesn't reach our gut microbes, however, they become less abundant, less diverse, and even begin to consume the mucus layer that protects the gut lining.

So, by thinking not only about ourselves when we choose our meals, but also about our microbes, we can improve our health and boost our happiness. Fiber is the nutrient they are after, and it is plants that we must eat to provide them with it. Whole grains, beans and peas, tubers, fruits, and vegetables all contribute to our fiber intake, whereas meat and other animal products are devoid of fiber altogether. Of course, to increase the amount of fiber each of us consumes, we need to make room on our plates. Reducing our meat intake, whether by having a smaller portion at each meal, or through the occasional plant-based meal, allows us to eat not just for ourselves, but for our 100 trillion friends.

HOW TO SATISFY YOUNG FUSSY EATERS

■ Ginny Messina

Author of *Vegan for Her: The Woman's Guide to Being Healthy and Fit on a Plant-Based Diet*

Introducing your family to menus that emphasize more plant foods can open up a world of possibilities for healthy and fun meals and snacks. As you explore meatless menu options, you'll have the opportunity to sample new foods from different cultures. You'll also discover new ways of meeting nutrient needs that can make your child's diet even more nutritious.

START THE DAY WITH A HEALTHFUL—AND FAMILIAR—BREAKFAST

Breakfast is simple if your child already likes cereal with milk. Opt for cereals that are lower in sugar and give them extra sweetness by topping with strawberries or sliced bananas. Serving cereal with vitamin C–rich foods like orange juice can improve absorption of the iron in the cereal. This is an especially important consideration for toddlers who are at risk for iron deficiency regardless of what type of diet they eat.

If your child enjoys it, soymilk is a great choice to pour over hot or cold cereal. Some research suggests that young girls who consume soy foods have a lower lifelong risk for breast cancer.

Children also love smoothies. Make them with frozen bananas and other fruit for a nutritious treat that is perfect for breakfast or a snack. Add silken tofu for a smoothie that is packed with protein.

SANDWICHES AND MORE FOR MEATLESS LUNCHES

If your child takes lunch to school, invest in some BPA-free plastic containers and a couple of wide-mouth thermal jars along with a thermal lunch bag. Fill a thermos with hot soup or veggie franks and beans. Pack a selection of raw vegetables or sliced apples with hummus or other bean spreads. Hearty salads made from whole grains with chopped nuts and celery added for crunch are another healthy option. Barley, brown rice, and couscous are mild-flavored grains that many children like.

Sandwich options include baked tofu, peanut or almond butter, and veggie burgers (store bought or homemade). Or try a no-tuna salad with mashed chickpeas combined with mayonnaise and chopped celery. Nut patés also make an appealing sandwich spread.

KID-PLEASING MEATLESS DINNERS

If your child's favorite dinner is a hamburger and French fries, then a bowl of lentil soup may not cut it. As you introduce younger family members to more meatless meals, it's helpful to begin with dishes that are similar to what they already enjoy. Try one of these simple meals:

- Veggie burger, baked "fries," cole slaw
- Tacos made with meatless ground "beef" and topped with chopped tomatoes and lettuce
- Macaroni and cheese (try making a cheesy sauce with soaked cashews for a healthy and delicious version of this comforting favorite), steamed broccoli, or carrots
- Pizza topped with lots of sautéed veggies
- Spaghetti and marinara sauce with veggie meatballs
- Peppers or tomatoes stuffed with a combination of brown rice, celery and walnuts

BEANS AND GREENS FOR CHILDREN

Leafy green veggies can be excellent sources of calcium, and they have a few other bone-building nutrients that your child won't get from milk. Most kids aren't crazy about kale, though. If you'd like to include some of these less common vegetables in your family's meals, consider a gentle introduction. Chop cooked kale into brown rice or any grain your child enjoys. Season with a dash of cinnamon and a sprinkle of salt, and roll in a tortilla.

Ideally, as you eat less meat, you'll eat more beans, which are among the most nutritious and health-promoting foods. But beans are relatively unfamiliar to many American adults and they are that much more so for kids. It is interesting, though, that some research shows many children enjoy beans. The two most popular dishes are chili and baked beans.

When first introducing them to young children, consider pairing beans with something sweet. White beans like navy or cannellini beans can be combined with chopped apples or figs.

Roasted chickpeas are another fun way to get kids to eat beans. Rinse and drain canned chickpeas and then toss them with a little tamari, lemon juice, and a teaspoon of maple syrup. Bake on a cookie sheet at 400°F for twenty to thirty minutes. These make a great finger food for a snack.

Canned or well-cooked navy beans can also be pureed into a sauce and served over grains or tossed with pasta for a protein-packed meal. It can take some experimenting to get children to eat beans, and it may take some time. But, while they may seem unusual to American kids, children throughout the world eat beans from infancy. An early introduction to these foods—even if it is small amounts and only occasionally—can set your child up for lifelong eating habits that help protect against chronic disease.

SNACK TIME FOR CHILDREN

Children, especially young ones, need snacks throughout the day. Keep healthy choices on hand to make the most of these mini-meals. They can be an easy way to set your mind at ease about whether your child is getting enough protein because some favorites are protein rich. Some good snack ideas for kids who are eating more plant foods include these:

- Trail mix with almonds, pumpkin seeds, and dried fruit
- Nutty fruit bites: dried fruit, nuts, and peanut or almond butter blended in a food processor and rolled into bite-size balls
- Soy nuts
- Homemade granola bars
- Homemade pancakes made with chickpea flour for a protein boost
- Chocolate tofu pudding
- Pinwheels: mix together hummus and shredded carrots and spread over a large whole wheat tortilla. Roll it up and slice into pinwheel rounds.

Helping children shift toward a diet that is lower in meat takes some trial and error and, of course, patience. But as you explore the options in this essay—and come up with some of your own ideas—you'll find there are plenty of meatless meals to please even the youngest palate.

THE MEAT LOBBY, THE POLITICIANS, AND U.S. NUTRITION

■ Jeffrey Sachs

Author of *The Price of Civilization: Reawakening American Virtue and Prosperity*

That U.S. politics is in the hands of the corporate lobbies is hardly news. Yet the brazen power of the lobbies, and the subservience of the politicians to them, is still a marvel to behold. We are familiar with the lobbying power of big oil, the military-industrial complex, the gun industry, the health insurers, and Wall Street. Yet in 2015 we watched the meat lobby undermine America's nutrition and food security, while the Obama administration dutifully fell into line.

Every five years the U.S. government puts out dietary guidelines based on the recommendations of the high-level Dietary Guidelines Advisory Committee of the nation's top nutrition experts. The goal is to review the scientific evidence to develop "food-based recommendations of public health importance for Americans age two years and older," according to the congressional testimony of U.S. Secretary of Agriculture Thomas Vilsack.

The 2015 Advisory Committee Report, written by a star-studded panel of scientific leaders, was notable for its insights into the linkages between nutrition, diet, and environmental sustainability, especially in Part D, Chapter 5, "Food Sustainability and Safety." The committee noted that the linkages between nutrition and food sustainability are crucial for the nutrition, food security, and public health of future generations of Americans. The committee also noted that many other countries—including Germany, Sweden, Netherlands, Australia, and Brazil—are already incorporating the linkages between nutrition and environment into nutritional recommendations.

The recommendations were built squarely on the *2010 Dietary*

Guidelines for Americans (DGA) report, which had already noted the need to take into account the sustainability of the diet with attention to future generations. The 2010 guidelines recognized the need to "Develop and expand safe, effective, and sustainable agriculture and aquaculture practices to ensure availability of recommended amounts of healthy foods to all segments of the population." The 2010 guidelines also recognized the intergenerational nature of the challenge: "By working together through policies, programs, and partnerships, we can improve the health of the current generation and take responsibility for giving future generations a better chance to lead healthy and productive lives."

In this spirit, the 2015 Advisory Committee determined that

> Consistent evidence indicates that, in general, a dietary pattern that is higher in plant-based foods, such as vegetables, fruits, whole grains, legumes, nuts, and seeds, and lower in animal-based foods is more health promoting and is associated with lesser environmental impact (GHG [greenhouse gas] emissions and energy, land, and water use) than is the current average U.S. diet. A diet that is more environmentally sustainable than the average U.S. diet can be achieved without excluding any food groups.

Note the appealing finding of synergy. Eating more vegetables and less meat is not only healthier but also environmentally more sustainable: a win-win conclusion.

This observation, nonetheless, is heresy, at least if you are a member of the meat lobby. A diet higher in vegetables, fruits, whole grains, legumes, nuts, and seeds, and lower in animal-based foods . . . those are fighting words. Indeed, the meat lobby swung into action, not by directly rejecting the committee's scientific findings, which it could not do, but by rejecting the role of the advisory committee in discussing the environmental impact of a meat-based diet.

The North American Meat Institute (NAMI), an industry body, declared the advisory committee unqualified to meddle in this area and the topic of environmental sustainability beyond the committee's scope: "The Committee's foray into the murky waters of sustainability is well beyond its scope and expertise. It's akin to having a dermatologist provide recommendations about cardiac care." It is not surprising that the NAMI did not call for corroborating evidence by additional environmental authorities but rather called for the U.S. Department of Agriculture (USDA) and Congress to quash the evidence by leaving Chapter 5 out of the final report.

It was at this stage that the secretary of agriculture added some notably apropos commentary to the U.S. political scene. In response to the advisory committee's ruthless, brazen attack on the meat interests, Secretary Vilsack had this to say: "[The] folks who put those reports together . . . have freedom. They are like my three-year-old granddaughter. She does not have to color inside the lines." His five-year-old grandson, by contrast, "is learning about coloring within the lines. I am going to color inside the lines." In short, environmental sustainability should play no part in the nutrition recommendations . . . especially, if it endangers the meat industry.

I admire Secretary Vilsack for his clarity in acknowledging that U.S. politics has descended to the level of five-year-olds. True to form, our childlike congressional representatives, dependent on largesse of the meat lobby, also weighed in to limit the scope of the nutrition guidelines, prompting the scientists to respond with a call to Congress for scientific objectivity and independence in the interests of America's public health.

At a time when the world is struggling to achieve an integrated vision of sustainable development; when the new Sustainable Development Goal 2 specifically calls on the world to "end hunger, achieve food security and improved nutrition, and promote sustainable agriculture"; and when climate change puts future food security at risk, the U.S. secretary of agriculture insists that America's top nutrition scientists should not examine the relationship between diet and environmental sustainability.

Of course there was a firestorm following Secretary Vilsack's admonition to the advisory committee to color within the lines and the attendant congressional meddling in the scientific work. Scientists, NGOs, and the public posted statements and filed petitions. Yet it was to no avail. On October 6, Secretary Vilsack and Health and Human Services Secretary Sylvia Burwell published a blog post making clear that environmental sustainability would not be part of the 2015 guidelines: "The final 2015 Guidelines are still being drafted, but because this is a matter of scope, we do not believe that the 2015 DGAs [Dietary Guidelines for Americans] are the appropriate vehicle for this important policy conversation about sustainability."

American politics is indeed broken. America's boosters will say, but yes, America is still number one. Alas, America is number one in the world in obesity, in carbon emissions per person (among large economies), and in income inequality in the high-income world. These ills are all of a piece: They reflect the subordination of the common interest to the corporate lobbies. But times will change, and scientific truth and decency will yet prevail; the American public is on to the corruption and cravenness of its elected officials.

FROM COMPULSIVE EATING TO CONSCIOUS EATING

■ Victoria Moran

Author of *Main Street Vegan: Everything You Need to Know to Eat Healthfully and Live Compassionately in the Real World* and *The Good Karma Diet: Eat Gently, Feel Amazing, Age in Slow Motion*

My name is Victoria and I am, in the interest of full disclosure, a vegan. It reminds me of the old commercial for deodorant soap that asked "Aren't you glad you use Dial? Don't you wish everybody did?" I am happy that I live and eat as I do and, yes, for a long list of reasons, I wish everybody did. I'm also aware that becoming vegan is, for most people, about on par with becoming Amish—admirable in many ways, but extreme, unusual, and culturally alien. I get it, because I'm a vegan now, but I wasn't always.

I grew up in Kansas City on its eponymous steak and barbecue. I loved animals the way most children do, bringing in every stray dog and cat, and attempting to save injured birds and orphaned baby squirrels, naive efforts that often ended in a backyard funeral.

I also had a strong interest in nutrition because my dad was a diet doctor and I was a fat kid. I read in one of his med school textbooks, when I was no more than nine, that the most nutrient-dense foods were collards, kale, mustard greens, arugula, Swiss chard, and spinach—that last entry being the only one I'd ever heard of, let alone tasted, and the spinach had come from a can.

Even earlier, I recall returning home from first grade and reciting the four food groups, the dietetic gold standard of the day, to my grandmother. Not one to readily accept government-sanctioned doctrine, she snorted, "Some people never eat meat. They're called vegetarians. I could take you to a certain restaurant and get you a hamburger made out of peanuts. You'd think you were eating beef."

She never took me to this curious café, but that word, *vegetarian*, struck a chord. I adored food in all its forms and presentations, so the idea that someone would cut out an entire "food group" was shocking. *I* certainly wasn't going to do it, but I found it intriguing that some people did. Gandhi had been vegetarian, I learned later— and Tolstoy and da Vinci. But they were famous and men and grown-ups. I was a girl from Kansas City.

It was an interest in yoga, which developed in my teens, and a move to veg-friendly London for a fashion course after high school, that inspired my initial change. I didn't know the term *reducetarian*, but that's what I was, letting go of poultry and red meat when I was eighteen, and fish at nineteen, although I had fishy relapses off and on. I didn't see water-dwelling animals as having self-awareness and feeling pain. Contemporary science contends that I was profoundly wrong on that, but at the time I was more interested in magic than science, and fish were said to hold some weight loss magic. It made no sense, then, that I kept getting bigger.

In my mid-twenties, a wise friend told me that I wasn't just randomly heavy. "You're a compulsive overeater," she said. "You'd stop if you could, but left to your own devices, you can't." Her words soaked in the way a houseplant takes up water when you get back from vacation.

Of course I'd stop if I could. I knew that. I'd do a lot of things. I wouldn't just be a vegetarian: I'd be a vegan, that steel-willed oddity who wouldn't drink milk or eat cheese because lactation requires pregnancy, and dairy calls for the separation of mother and babe and the ultimate slaughter of both. Yes! Count me on the side of the weird and valiant. I will do this.

But I didn't. I couldn't make it to lunch at work most days without a trip to the office building's snack bar where I wasn't thinking of cows and calves, but of a craving for ice cream or a pastry rich in butter and eggs. Some people say food isn't a real addiction. I know different.

Like any other addict—any lucky addict—I stumbled onto recovery: take some steps, have a spiritual awakening, do it a day at a time. It sounds cliché in some circles, and more religious than rational, but after thirty-two years without a binge, it works for me. It gave me the power of choice around food, and once I had that, I chose vegan. I wasn't perfect. This was a long time ago, when eating out as a vegan was tough and traveling seemed close to impossible. I sometimes didn't ask what was in a prepared item that may have been vegan or maybe only vegetarian. But I kept at it. In time, choosing vegan on a consistent basis became easy and natural, and even when it wasn't, animal products didn't seem like food anymore, just like sadness.

So, should you reduce your consumption of animal foods or go vegan? Well, what are you willing to do? If you're over fifty and terms like *heart attack*, *stroke*, and *Alzheimer's* seem less theoretical than they once did, I'd suggest going all the way simply to lower your anxiety level. My diet today, in my sixties, is a feast of age-defraying antioxidants and disease-preventing phytochemicals from whole plant foods. If I'm offered a vegan cookie, I may eat it, although I'd prefer a kiwi or a mango that will actually do something in addition to taste good.

But you know what? Most of the plant-based experts contend that, health wise, 90 percent whole plant foods should do you.

Ethically, every little bit helps. Not a single plant-sourced meal fails to contribute to lives saved and suffering averted. Don't let yourself be guilt tripped into doing nothing by the vegan police, amnesiacs who can't recall that they were once where you are right now.

On the other hand, be aware that the day may dawn when you realize that you've developed vegan values. This is the day you see a piece of chicken for what it is: part of a bird. This is when a carton of yogurt is less about calcium and convenience than a mother cow and her baby crying in the grief of separation. (Calcium, by the way, is abundant in dark leafy greens, nondairy milks, and calcium-cultured tofu.) Just as you stood up to the vegan police before, hold your own with the omnivore army now. They'll ask where you get your protein (answer: from whole plant foods) and suggest that animals may take over the world (they won't; we breed them). You have every right to eat as you wish and live as you choose. If these choices happen to enrich your life and save many others, so much the better.

THE CHALLENGE OF FEEDING LESS MEAT TO DOGS AND CATS

■ Pete Wedderburn

Veterinary surgeon and author of *My Dog Thinks He's Human* and *My Cat Is Ignoring Me!*

Many vegans and vegetarians are also animal lovers, and they struggle with the fact that standard pet foods often contain meat of unknown origin. Is there any way around this? Can dogs and cats eat less or no meat?

The answer for dogs is straightforward enough, mostly because dogs are such omnivores. A 2013 study demonstrated that over 10,000 years ago, around the time that dogs first were becoming domesticated, they developed the digestive apparatus (anatomy and enzymes) needed to digest plant-sourced starches as well as meat.[1] This means that as long their food is prepared with the correct amount of protein (including specific amino acids), carbohydrates, oils, vitamins, and minerals, dogs are perfectly capable of eating vegetarian, or even vegan. A 2009 study proved that even hardworking, sled-pulling Huskies were able to thrive on a balanced, meat-free diet.[2]

The safest way for pet owners to implement this kind of a diet is to seek out commercially manufactured vegetarian or vegan dog food that has already demonstrated its efficacy in scientific trials. Such products are legally obliged to fulfill specific nutritional criteria, formulated by professional nutritionists. If the label states that the dog food is "complete," it means the chow has been formulated to meet the dietary needs of your dog. While it's theoretically possible to prepare vegetarian dog food from scratch, the recipe is tricky. You would need to engage the services of a professional nutritionist to ensure the formula you created was adequate. To be safe, you might even need to ask your vet for regular blood tests to ensure your dog's metabolism was running properly. Given these challenges, most dog owners find commercially produced vegetarian dog food is the most cost-efficient and risk-free option.

Dog owners, it turns out, have it easy. It's far more difficult for cats to go vegetarian or vegan. Cats are known as "obligate carnivores." Their biological structure—from their teeth to their digestive tract and metabolism rates—have all evolved to efficiently process a typical diet of small prey animals. While a cat's anatomy can digest plant-based food when necessary, a few critical aspects of the feline metabolism require nutrients that are commonly found only in meat. Other mammals do not have this requirement; it's an exclusively feline characteristic.

Compared to dogs, cats have a high protein requirement because of different enzyme pathways. They also require specific amino acids, including one, taurine, that occurs naturally only in meat. (It can be synthetically manufactured from chemicals of nonmeat origin, however.) Taurine deficiency causes serious illness in cats, such as fatal heart disease, so pet food manufacturers must be certain their products contain sufficient quantities.

Cats also require an amino acid called arginine. While most common in meat, the amino acid can be found in specific plant sources. Arginine is needed for daily protein synthesis as well as for ammonia detoxification; a cat being fed a plant-based diet without enough arginine will rapidly develop signs of ammonia toxicity. There is almost no risk of this happening when cats eat a meat-based diet. Similarly, cats require arachidonic acid, an essential fatty acid that is, once again, found commonly only in animal tissue. Deficiencies here can cause problems with fat metabolism, abnormal blood clotting, and skin disease. Cats on a meat-free diet will need special supplements to ensure they get enough of this essential nutrient. They will also need a preformed version of vitamin A, which is found naturally only in meat, and vitamin B_{12}, which they would otherwise ingest with animal tissue. Synthetic supplements are available for these vitamins as well, but must be given carefully and in the correct quantities.

If cats do not get all of their essential nutrients, they may become ill or even die prematurely. So while it's possible to feed cats on a vegetarian or vegan diet, cat owners need to factor in the risks before forcing a meat-eating animal to eat a diet its body was not originally designed to consume. If owners feel comfortable making this decision, they need to research and formulate the new diet carefully, preferably while working under the guidance of a nutritional specialist (a member of the American College of Veterinary Nutrition or European College of Veterinary and Comparative Nutrition).

Once the proper diet has been agreed on, owners should test their cat's urine once a month to make sure it's sufficiently acidic. Plant-based diets can cause alkaline urine, which in turn can cause dangerous urinary tract obstructions, especially in male cats. Furthermore, a twice-yearly visit to the veterinarian for a full physical examination is the best way to check for signs of nutrient excess or deficiency.

As with any diet, owners should pick only commercial nonmeat cat foods that have been sufficiently tested by the manufacturer. Unfortunately, to my knowledge, no vegan or vegetarian cat food manufacturer has yet done this. An Australian company did commission a short, unpublished study on protein digestibility and palatability for both vegan dogs and cats. But the study in question did not meet the Association of American Feed Control Officials (AAFCO) guidelines, an international benchmark of acceptability.

The bottom line for reducetarian dog and cat owners? It's much easier to switch your dog over to a non-meat-based diet, and there are plenty of manufacturer-tested, commercially available food options to choose from. But any change in your pet's diet needs to be evaluated carefully and the risks weighed against the benefits. The safest option may be to simply reduce the meat in your pet's diet—but even with this compromise, the overall nutritional composition of the diet must remain the same. When in doubt, consult with a nutritional specialist—never assume a random, "sensible" mix of meat and vegetables will be sufficient. This is particularly important for cats, which can suffer significantly if their unique nutritional needs are not met. Ultimately, choosing a more humane, meat-based cat food may be the most practical compromise for cat owners wishing to minimize animal cruelty.

WHAT CHAMPION ATHLETES EAT TO STAY ON TOP OF THEIR GAME

Gene Baur

President of Farm Sanctuary and author of *Living The Farm Sanctuary Life: The Ultimate Guide to Eating Mindfully, Living Longer, and Feeling Better Every Day*

We grow up being told that meat and other animal products are nutritious and necessary for building strong bodies and fueling athletic performance. But the fact is, due to plants' high carbohydrate, low fat, and protein-rich composition, we can live well and maintain a high athletic standard while eating a plant-based diet.

Fruit, vegetables, whole grains, and legumes have fueled athletes for centuries. Indeed, 2,000 years ago, Roman gladiators endured grueling training schedules on a vegetarian diet. Fast-forward a few millennia, and plenty of modern-day fighters still swear by a plant-based regimen. In the film *Forks over Knives*, mixed martial arts (MMA) fighter Mac Danzig extolls the benefits of plant-based nutrition on camera. Other successful fighters who adhere to similar nutrition plans include Ultimate Fighting Champion (UFC) heavyweight Mark Hunt, heavyweight boxer and 2016 Olympian Cam Awesome, and welterweight boxing champion Timothy Bradley, who ended the legendary Manny Pacquiao's seven-year undefeated streak in 2012.

Plant-fueled athletes have also succeeded at the highest levels of endurance, strength, and speed competitions. Scott Jurek is a legendary endurance runner and ultra-marathon champion, who won the 100-mile Western States Endurance Run seven times as a vegan. Meanwhile, vegan strongman Patrik Baboumian set a Guinness World Record in 2015 by carrying more than 1,200 pounds for ten meters.

Still, animal products remain front and center at many sporting events and fill the pages of fitness publications. Various industries maintain marketing agreements with sporting and health organizations, and may even sponsor competitions. After finishing several marathons and triathlons, I've had to politely turn down containers of cow's milk thrust on athletes at the finish line by well-meaning volunteers.

There is plenty of truth to the old adage, We are what we eat; our food gives us energy, which is then incorporated into the cells of our bodies. Of course, eating an ox won't make you as strong as one—ironically, oxen derive much of their strength from eating plants. Science is on my side here, and many health and nutrition experts have spent years trying to debunk the idea that animal products are a key component of athletic preparation.

Over the past decade, these voices of reason have increased substantially in both numbers and volume. Take Brendan Brazier, a Canadian 50K ultra-marathon champion, who has spent years perfecting his own plant-based nutrition supplement called Vega. Brazier has consulted as a trainer for Hollywood celebrities as well as a wide range of professional athletes. But Brazier is just the tip of the iceberg. With growing awareness about the myriad health problems associated with animal-heavy diets, more and more citizens are learning firsthand the benefits of reducing everyday meat consumption. If you're an athlete looking to incorporate some extra plant-based protein into your diet, here are a few simple tips to help get you started:

- Mix chickpeas, kidney beans, and black beans into your salad. These legumes have as much as 10 grams of protein per serving.
- Blend almond, soy, or cashew milk into your favorite fresh or frozen fruits for a thick and creamy high-protein shake. (Fun fact: Soy milk has the highest protein count of all non-dairy milks, equal to the protein found in a same-size serving of cow's milk.)
- Accompany vegetable stir-fries with quinoa, a grain loaded with around 6 grams of protein per serving.
- Supercharge your morning with a firm or extra-firm tofu scramble breakfast. Extra-firm tofu is a complete protein, meaning it contains the nine essential amino acids the body needs to help maintain muscle, bone, and organs.
- Remember, veggies and fruits can themselves be valuable sources of protein—1 cup of cooked spinach has nearly 5 grams. Popeye was on to something after all.

THE OMEGA-3 PARADOX: HOW WE BECAME DEFICIENT IN THE MOST ABUNDANT FAT ON THE PLANET

■ Susan Allport

Author of *The Queen of Fats: Why Omega-3s Were Removed from the Western Diet and What We Can Do to Replace Them*

Have you ever wondered why Americans—who, like all humans, evolved on the savannas of Africa—are now being advised to consume fish twice a week?

This would boost our consumption of omega-3s, of course, essential fats that are important for the health of our hearts and brains and every other tissue in the body. But how did we come to be deficient in these fast-acting fats? And where did early humans on the savannas get their daily dose of omega-3s?

Now some would argue that fish have always been a mainstay of the human diet and that this ancient food choice is in fact responsible for the evolution of our large brains.

But there's a simpler explanation—one that doesn't require any revisions to the archaeological record. It begins with the fact that omega-3s don't originate in fish, but rather in the chloroplasts of green leaves, including plankton, the green leaves of the oceans.

The parent omega-3, alpha-linolenic acid, is found in highest concentrations in the membranes of the chloroplasts of green leaves. And because green leaves are the most abundant thing on the planet, it follows that omega-3s are the most abundant fat. They're not the rare nutrient we've been led to believe. They're all around us and in most of our foods.

Alpha-linolenic acid helps plants photosynthesize—capture light molecules and turn them into sugars—the basis, need I say it, of all life on earth. Photosynthesis is a plant's speediest and most metabolically demanding activity, requiring the coordination of about seventy-five different enzymes. Alpha-linolenic acid, a fat with three kinks (or double bonds) in its structure, enables all those enzymes to run quickly and smoothly.

Animals that eat green leaves accumulate lots of this speedy omega-3 fat in their tissues. But because animals are faster—that is, more mobile—than plants they make this fat even speedier (kinkier) by adding length and double bonds to its structure. Animals then concentrate those elongated fats (known as DHA and EPA) in their most metabolically active tissue: their brains, hearts, eyes, and muscles, including the muscle of the heart.

For most of human history, humans never had a problem consuming enough omega-3s. There was no such thing as an omega-3 deficiency. Our ancestors would have gotten this essential nutrient from the many plants and greens they ate. Or via the eggs they foraged and the animals they hunted, animals that had themselves consumed plants and greens. For most of human history, heart disease and all the other ailments linked to a deficiency of omega-3s were rare phenomena. Fish wouldn't have added much in the way of omega-3s to most diets.

But all that changed at the beginning of the twentieth century when Americans began to consume more and more seeds, and especially seed oils, a trend that began in the early 1900s with the first commercial presses for extracting oil from seeds. (Before then, butter and lard were the most common added fats.) And when farmers began feeding the animals they raised on seeds instead grass, a method of husbandry that was fueled by the corn surpluses of the post–World War II era.

Seeds, such as corn and soybeans, are much richer in a second family of essential fats: omega-6s, which we now know compete with omega-3s for positions in our cell membranes and have very different effects on membranes and health. Omega-6s promote blood clotting, inflammation, tumor growth, and weight gain while omega-3s protect against all these. We need both omega-3s and omega-6s in our diets and our tissues, but because they compete with each other for a limited number of positions in cell membranes, too many omega-6s causes a deficiency of omega-3s. It's like a game of musical chairs. There are only so many chairs in the game, and if they are occupied by omega-6s, they can't be occupied by omega-3s.

Let's look at a few foods to see just how omega-6s out-compete omega-3s. Say you decide to eat the greenest, healthiest lunch possible—a big bowl of steamed spinach. It doesn't have much fat in it but the fat there is are mostly omega-3s (true of any bowl of greens)—until you dress it with a modest tablespoon or so of peanut . . . or grape-seed . . . or sesame oil dressing. Now, suddenly, that once healthful bowl of spinach has at least ten times the omega-6s as omega-3s. Only a concentrated source of omega-3s, such as a piece of fish, could offset this unfortunate turn of events.

Because fish live under pressure in cold, dim environments, they require more omega-3s in their diet and tissues than terres-trial animals—and are indeed a great source of these vital, flexible fats. But there aren't enough fish in the ocean to fix America's omega-6 habit this way. Americans would have to eat about ten times as much fish as they currently do to meet current recommen-dations. And most of our fisheries are already overstressed.

If, on the other hand, Americans simply consumed less omega-6s, by choosing oils and fats that have a better balance to begin with—canola, for example, a seed oil that happens to have a very healthy balance of omega-3s and omega-6s (and, yes, there are non-GMO canola oils!), or a mixture of canola and olive—and by greatly reduc-ing their consumption of corn- and soy-fed meats, eggs, and dairy, there would be no need for the fish solution. Other oils that have a healthy balance are flax and hemp seed oils, which shouldn't be used for cooking but can be added to dressings.

This is not the first time populations have created a nutritional deficiency with their agricultural techniques—think of the epidem-ics of beriberi in the nineteenth century when Asian populations relied on polished white rice, stripped of its vitamin B_1-bearing husk—as a staple food. And it probably won't be the last. But how we solve our omega-3 deficiency matters greatly, not just for our in-dividual health, but for the health of our oceans—and the fish that swim them.

HOW TO LIVE LONG AND DIE WELL

■ Gene Stone

Author of *The Secrets of People Who Never Get Sick: What They Know, Why It Works, and How It Can Work for You*

In 2013, a study of more than 73,000 subjects by researchers at Loma Linda University in California created compelling headlines around the world. According to the report, vegetarians had a 12 percent lower risk of dying over a six-year period than nonvegetarians. Vegans had even better numbers: a 15 percent lower risk of death. (Lacto-ovo vegetarians, who consume dairy and eggs, had a 9 percent lower risk, and semi-vegetarians, who eat some meat, had an 8 percent lower risk.)

As remarkably cheerful as plant-based eaters found this news, there's more to consider. For one, vegetarians and vegans in general tend to be more health conscious and thinner than the general population. So perhaps it wasn't their diet as much as other facets of their daily life that kept the subjects alive. Furthermore, the Loma Linda subjects weren't exactly your average cola-guzzling, burger-gobbling Americans: All of them belonged to the Seventh-day Adventist Church, whose health-conscious members do not drink liquor or smoke cigarettes. They don't even drink coffee. They don't even drink tea. In fact, Loma Linda, home to one of the largest Adventist congregations in the world, is the only American city that qualifies as a Blue Zone. Blue zones, discovered by author Dan Buettner, are locations where inhabitants live unusually long and healthy lives. Finally, vegan diets haven't been around long enough for anyone to be able to prove that plant-based eaters enjoy longer life spans than carnivores. Come back in another generation or two, people say, and the science will be clearer.

However, there are other highly encouraging signs that plant-based eating has significant health benefits. A whole-food vegan diet is very low in cholesterol and saturated fats and high in fiber and complex carbohydrates, all of which lead to better health. Plant-based eaters tend to have a much higher frequency of bowel movements, which is also strongly associated with better health. Vegans have been shown to have lower levels of inflammation than those who consume animal protein—another marker of good health.

There's more: Eating a plant-based diet has been strongly associated with lower blood levels of industrial pollutants than an omnivorous diet. The breast milk of vegans has been found to be significantly less polluted with fire retardants and dioxins than that of meat-eating moms. Mercury levels in vegans have also been found to be ten times lower than in those who eat fish. Consider that because Americans feed farm animals to other farm animals, the toxins in these creatures' bodies bioaccumulate up the food chain before the meat lands on an omnivore's plate. So eating lower on the food chain (a plant-based diet) may decrease exposure to the industrial pollutants linked to poor health.

Despite the myth that vegans don't get enough calcium, plant-based eaters have been found to have bone density similar to omnivores', and vegans even have been found to have higher blood-plasma protein levels than meat eaters. An egg-free vegetarian diet has also been found to result in higher blood levels of the hormone DHEA, which may extend one's lifespan. Vegans also appear to be at the lowest risk for developing arthritis and cataracts. Rheumatoid arthritis can in some cases be reversed by a vegan diet. A plant-based diet also appears to prevent and even treat Crohn's disease. And plant-based diets may prevent kidney function decline and possibly treat kidney failure.

In fact, a plant-based diet has been shown to help prevent or reverse the fifteen leading causes of death in America, which claim 1.6 million lives annually. In his recent book *How Not to Die*, Dr. Michael Greger, director of Public Health and Animal Agriculture at the Humane Society of America,[1] shows how a plant-based diet can prevent or reverse: coronary heart disease, lung disease, brain disease, digestive cancers, infections, diabetes, high blood pressure, liver disease, blood cancers, kidney disease, breasts cancer, suicidal depression, prostate cancer, Parkinson's disease, and iatrogenic disease (conditions caused by medications and other medical treatments).

Furthermore, the newest research on telomeres seems to corroborate Dr. Greger's research. Telomeres are the caps on the ends of our DNA strands that protect our chromosomes, akin to the aglets at the end of shoelaces. Our telomeres need to stay as intact as possible because shortening affects our health and, quite possibly, our lifespan.

The first telomere studies were published in the 1970s (one of the principal researchers, Elizabeth Blackburn, shared the 2009 Nobel Prize in Medicine for this work). A more recent study from the University of California, San Francisco, indicated that men who switched to a vegetarian diet were able to protect their telomeres, thus enhancing their health. Another study, published in the journal *Lancet Oncology*, showed that a plant-based, whole-foods vegan diet, along with stress management, exercise, and social support, backed up previous studies that found participants' telomeres were longer and stronger.[2] That research was overseen by Dr. Dean Ornish, founder and president of the Preventive Medical Research Institute and clinical professor of medicine at the university.

Not all scientists are convinced that longer telomeres are indeed a marker of longevity, although a 2012 study from the University of East Anglia supports Ornish's findings. The researchers wrote, "We saw that telomere length is a better indicator of life expectancy than chronological age." So did an announcement made by Salt Lake City's Intermountain Heart Institute at the American College of Cardiology's Annual Scientific Session: "Our research shows that if we statistically adjust for age, patients with longer telomeres live longer, suggesting that telomere length is more than just a measure of age."

Convincing stuff. But not proof. The jury will be out until medical science has had the opportunity to conduct research on multiple generations of vegans, vegetarians, and semi-vegetarians. However, these studies do suggest that even if the life spans of vegans and omnivores turn out to be comparable, those who ate more plant-based meals and fewer animal products will have enjoyed better health throughout their lives.

Think of it this way: Which would you rather do—live nine healthy decades and then die quickly, and or live the same number of mostly disease-ridden years? It's not necessarily how long we live, but how well we die.

FALL IN LOVE WITH PLANTS

Sharon Palmer

The Plant-Powered Dietitian, author of *Plant-Powered for Life* and *The Plant-Powered Diet*

Fall in love with plants and they will love you back. That's one of my favorite sayings whenever I find myself talking about the power of a plant-based eating style. It may sound painfully obvious, but in today's chaotic world we're so removed from the source of plant foods—that is the living plant with its roots dug into the soil—that it's difficult to see the "plant" for the forest. It's hard to imagine a cornstalk with bulging ears of corn rustling in the wind when you peer into a bag of corn chips. And it's hard to recall the sweet perfume from a row of ripe strawberry plants when you're downing strawberry-flavored yogurt. And thanks to so many confusing nutrition messages—carbs are bad, avoid grains—plant foods have lost their healing power for so many people. Yet every edible plant—bulb, tuber, leaf, stalk, seed, flower, and fleshy orb we call fruit—has a nourishing story to tell.

Humans and plants have long lived together in harmony—each helping the other along the road to survival. For example, fruits evolved their tantalizing sweet flesh encasing seeds as a mere means of attracting animals and humans to pluck the fruit, spit out the seeds, and thus disperse them for the next generation. In return, the plants bestowed on humans a wide range of powerful nutrients that helped not only to provide energy and sustenance but to protect health, too. Plants never had the ability to get up and run away from their environmental threats, such as the sun, pests, or disease. So they developed protective compounds—often concentrated in their peel or skin—to shield them from such threats. And it turns out that those compounds—which are often related to the color and flavor of the plant—protect us too.

Dark gem-like berries have anthocyanin compounds, which are good for the brain. Scarlet tomatoes have lycopene, which helps protect the skin. And those pungent sulfur compounds in cabbage and kale help fight cancer. Scientists are discovering new compounds in plants all the time. And it's not just limited to fruits and vegetables—there are protective compounds in all whole plant foods, including whole grains, such as wheat, quinoa, and barley; legumes, like beans and lentils; nuts, including almonds and walnuts; seeds, such as hemp and sunflower seeds; and even spices, herbs, tea, coffee, and chocolate.

No wonder that study after study finds that eating more whole plant foods is linked with a lower risk of heart disease, type 2 diabetes, and certain types of cancer. Even the Dietary Guidelines Advisory Committee—our nation's top nutrition experts tasked with coming up with recommendations for the best eating pattern for optimal health—suggests eating a plant-based diet.

The key to eating a plant-based diet for health is to eat those plants in their whole state—what I call "as close to the earth as possible." What I mean by that is that the food actually looks like part of the plant that grows in the soil—a leaf from a spinach plant, a kernel of farro from a grass plant, a sunflower seed from the center of a sunflower. Because if you really think about it, soda is a plant-based food and so is a giant white bagel. Yet it's hard to think of a single whole plant food growing in the soil when you down a soda or a big white bagel. Those ingredients may have come from plants, but they've been so processed and refined down from corn (corn syrup in the soda) and wheat (white flour in the bagel), they are a distant memory of the original plant. And now we know that eating foods in these highly processed forms isn't such a healthy habit. A plethora of research is rolling in on how sweetened beverages are linked with obesity and type 2 diabetes, and large amounts of refined grains have been called out for their role in obesity and cardiovascular risks.

The most beautiful benefit of a plant-based diet—by definition a diet that focuses on plants over animals—is not so much about what you don't eat; it's more about what you do eat. Plants! Research shows that people who eat a plant-based diet are eating sometimes two to three times the amounts of fruits, vegetables, whole grains, legumes, nuts, and seeds compared with the average person. That's why they tend to live longer, and have less heart disease, cancer, and diabetes. So instead of focusing on what you can't have as you shift your diet to plants, think more about what you can have.

There are more than 40,000 edible plant species on the planet, and each species has remarkable diversity with sometimes thousands of varieties. Just think of the amazing choices you have when you put plants at the center of your plate. You can feast on one of a thousand different varieties of tomatoes, such as Purple Cherokee, Green Zebra, and Golden Gem—each with its own amazing color, flavor, and texture. Or you can call on the earthy, nutrient-rich bean family—which consists of about 40,000 bean varieties—to replace meat at the dinner table. You can choose a mint green Flageolet, a fleshy red Calypso, or a small Yellow Indian Women bean to feature in a casserole, chili, or salad. And you can savor the most succulent ripe peach—whether a red-yellow Dessert Gold or a white-fleshed Snow Beauty variety. The choices are astonishing.

Which leads me to one more important thought on plant-based eating: It's not only healthful—it's downright delicious! A plate of meat can never capture the nuances, flavors, colors, and textures of plant foods. Just consider a wisp of a micro sprout, a crunchy enoki mushroom, a pungent leaf of red chard, a tart wedge of grapefruit, a sweet-spicy shred of ginger, and a creamy avocado slice. Many of our most beloved dishes from around the world focus on plants, whether it's spaghetti with a vibrant tomato-based sauce with herbs; a crisp corn tortilla filled with beans, cabbage, avocados, and tomatoes; or a stir-fry of crisp snow peas, onions, mushrooms, and ginger with rice. So, go ahead—fall in love with plants, and let them love you right back.

FOOD, REPRODUCTION, AND THE EVOLUTION OF THE HUMAN BODY

■ David Bainbridge

Anatomist and reproductive biologist at Cambridge University and author of several popular science books, including *Curvology: the Origin and Power of Female Body Shape*

We humans are a bizarre species. In the 7 or 8 million years since we diverged evolutionarily from the ancestors of our closest relatives, the chimpanzees and gorillas, we have undergone a series of exceptional and often unique biological and ecological innovations. As a result, the interactions among food, fertility, and body shape in humans are unlike those seen anywhere else in the animal kingdom.

Climate change is thought to have been a major stimulus for the evolution of our species. The human lineage appeared at a time when its native Africa was becoming more arid, forests were receding, and more open environments were starting to predominate. Why our ancestors switched from the more arboreal habitats of their ancestors and relatives and migrated to the open plains is uncertain, but the changes this wrought on our species' structure and biology were dramatic. Fossil evidence suggests that once humans were freed from the need to move swiftly though the forest canopy, they soon adapted to an entirely novel, bipedal form of locomotion. Human walking and running are impressively efficient processes, especially considering that no other animal has ever evolved anything similar. Our ancestors' limbs were effectively "back-engineered" to regain a "pre-primate" morphology not unlike that seen in modern-day bears, and the pelvis and lower spine underwent dramatic distortions to allow our upright stance.

Bipedalism soon led to other distinctive human adaptations,

and the most unusual of these was an increase in brain size. In general, the size of animals' brains exhibits a fairly reliable mathematical relationship to their body size, and few species deviate from this relationship. However, the human brain is approximately five times larger than would be expected of a mammal our size, and this is probably why humans are so intelligent. Most striking of all is the fact that, in all of evolutionary history, no other species has undergone such rapid and pronounced brain enlargement.

It is thought that the large human brain evolved when changes in our ancestors' environment drove them to adopt new modes of food acquisition. Humans are not especially strong, fast, or armed, yet around the world they have adapted to ecological niches that involve the acquisition of uncommon, hard-to-acquire, high-value food items. In times of environmental adversity, it is often humans who survive by excavating, picking, or removing the indigestible rind from nutritious plants or by killing and eating animals that are more swift or ferocious than themselves. This human focus on using sheer intelligence and communal cooperation to thrive is unparalleled in the animal kingdom. Perhaps the species most similar to us in this respect is the killer whale, and it is no surprise that humans and orcas now exhibit perhaps the widest geographical distribution of any mammalian species. However, while killer whales' high-value foodstuffs are entirely constituted by fish or meat, the question of the relative importance of plant and animal foods in human evolution remains an open one.

Indeed, traditional anthropological narratives tend to place hunting for meat at the center of human life and evolution, although this is increasingly viewed as scientific chauvinism—after all, in almost all human societies it is men who do most hunting, even though that hunting may contribute only a small proportion of their social group's nutritional needs. It has even been suggested that hunting for meat evolved as an unintended consequence of predator deterrence. According to this theory, our ancestors' upright stance freed their arms and hands for other activities, and one of those activities was fending off predators. The human hand, arm, and shoulder (especially in the male) are well adapted for throwing rocks and sticks at marauding animals that might otherwise consider puny upright apes to be easy pickings. The fortuitous discovery that throwing objects at predatory animals occasionally led to the death and potential eating of those animals may have spurred the refinement of these skills for deliberate hunting of prey species.

Thus the human evolutionary lineage is a continuing story of increased dependence on intelligence. However, the huge brain required to permit that intelligence itself places tremendous demands on our species. Brain tissue uses a large amount of energy, and the development of the human brain in fetal life represents an enormous burden on parental resources. Consider, for example, that a newborn baby generates 1 million new brain cells every twenty seconds, or that 85 percent of the energy used by a sleeping newborn is utilized in its brain. Unlike other mammalian species, the human brain continues to grow just as fast in the first few years of life as it did before birth, and most of the energy and nutrients to fuel that process must be supplied by the mother via breast milk. This drain on maternal resources is compounded by the fact that human offspring take an exceptionally long time to reach maturity, and that human mothers differ from most primates in that they often care simultaneously for multiple children of different ages.

It is these unique pressures on human mothers that lie behind the strikingly different body morphologies of the two sexes. When human babies are born, approximately 13 percent of their body weight is fat. By the end of puberty, the figure for boys remains around 13 percent, whereas for girls it has increased to 27 percent. Estrogenic drive during puberty causes the deposition of 10 to 12 kilograms (22 to 26 pounds) of adipose tissue in various locations around the body, but especially in the buttocks and thighs. And notably, this "gluteofemoral" fat is remarkably stable in the face of dietary restriction and is mobilized only after birth to supply the needs of the mammary glands as they produce copious lipid-rich milk to drive neonatal brain growth. Not only is fat high in calories, but the developing brain itself also needs specific lipid molecules—after water, fat is the largest constituent of the human brain. In other words, it is the uniquely human female curviness that has allowed our species to become so intelligent and successful.

All this leaves the question—what food types best support our species' energy-intensive, intelligence-driven, huge-brained lifestyle? There can be little doubt that our ancestors' nutritional needs were met by a combination of plant and animal foods. However, there is evidence from hunter-gatherer societies around the world that the relative contribution of meat and plants can vary greatly. It seems that the question is one of quantity of food, rather than exact type. As long as sufficient adipose stores have been established in mothers' thighs and buttocks, it seems to matter little whether the main food supply is largely vegetarian. Over most of human evolution, the environmental effects of meat eating by tiny human populations have been negligible, and few of our ancestors ate enough meat to suffer any pathological consequences. With the advent of agriculture approximately 10,000 years ago, and the more recent intensification of farming and consequent increase in the availability of meat, that situation has, of course, changed.

SEEKING THE OPTIMAL DIET TO MAXIMIZE DISEASE REVERSAL AND LONGEVITY

Joel Fuhrman

President of the Nutritional Research Foundation; board-certified family physician and nutritional researcher; author of five *New York Times* best sellers on superior nutrition, weight loss, and longevity

Food can be divided into four main categories; produce, whole grains, refined or highly processed foods, and animal products. Americans consume about 55 percent of calories from refined foods and approximately 30 percent of calories from animal products, with only about 15 percent of calories from a combination of whole grains and produce. This small amount of produce, especially greens, mushrooms, onions, seeds, colorful vegetables, and fruits, leads to an overall deficiency in micronutrients, especially antioxidants and phytochemicals necessary for normal health, cellular repair, and healthy immune function.

Animal products do not contain a significant micronutrient load compared to vegetables, and they are void of antioxidants and phytochemicals. It is well established that modest micronutrient insufficiency is ubiquitous and can lead to an increase in free radicals, inflammation, DNA damage, mitochondrial decay, and telomere decay, laying the foundation of disease and premature aging. If we classify phytochemicals as a form of micronutrients because of their relation to immune function, disease protection, and longevity, then we must classify almost all Americans (both vegetarians and meatatarians) as micronutrient deficient, especially regarding micronutrients derived from green vegetables.

Using the presence or absence of animal products as the distinguishing characteristic is a narrow and unsatisfactory way to characterize a diet designed to maximize health and disease reversal. A vegan diet is defined as one free of animal-based foods. A "plant-based" diet is often used in place of the word *vegan*, though the meaning of that term is questionable, especially considering that the word *based* is generally understood to mean the majority (over 50 percent). Even the standard American diet (SAD) with 30 percent of calories from animal products can be accurately called "plant-based."

A vegan diet may or may not be healthful depending on its design, and even when carefully designed, supplementation is necessary to ensure adequacy of all nutrients. Furthermore, the potential risk of consuming animal products can be largely obliterated by a reduction in their use, rather than a total elimination. There are multiple long-term studies that document reduction in both cardiovascular death (strokes and heart attacks) and cancer deaths in diets lower in animal products. The precise amount of animal products allowed to maximize prevention of disease and enhance longevity has not been determined.

It has become increasingly evident that higher levels of insulin-like growth factor 1 (IGF-1) are linked to increased early life mortality, higher incidence of cancer, and premature aging, including aging of the brain. It is also well established that diets with excessive amount of animal protein elevate IGF-1 and that optimally low levels are not achieved until a significant reduction in animal products is maintained in the diet. Eating more plant protein and less animal protein is a simple formula to extend the human lifespan. Studies generally demonstrate that above 5 to 10 percent of calories from animal products can raise IGF-1 significantly.[1]

I propose that, after reviewing the preponderance of evidence on these issues, the vast majority of informed nutritional scientists and physicians who have no predetermined agenda or bias would be forced to agree on these three dietary principles:

1. Vegetables, beans, seeds, nuts, and fruits are good for you.

2. Excessive amounts of animal products increase chronic disease risk.

3. Refined carbohydrates promote chronic disease and lead to overweight and obesity.

I have observed for more than twenty years that a diet designed around natural plant foods with the liberal use of greens, nuts, and beans has resulted in long-term sustained weight loss and reversal of high blood pressure, diabetes, and heart disease in thousands of overweight individuals. We surveyed 768 of these people, and tracked a reduction in their caloric drive and addictive sensations that drove overeating behavior in their past.[2] Those most adherent to the program had the most modified reduction in hunger.

Now is the time to take advantage of modern nutritional science. One thing we know for sure: The way Americans are eating today has resulted in a sickly, medically dependent society, with healthcare costs that are unsustainable and needless suffering and tragedies.

A DEADLY GAME OF TELEPHONE: FROM THE RESEARCH LAB TO YOUR FACEBOOK FEED

■ Howard Jacobson

Founder of TriangleBeWell.com and contributing author
to *Proteinaholic: How Our Obsession with Meat Is Killing Us
and What We Can Do About It* by Garth Davis, MD

One morning not so long ago, I woke up to find an unusual headline was going viral on my Facebook feed: "New Study Claims Eating Bacon May Prolong Your Life." It took me about ten minutes of clicking from blogs to newspapers to press releases to find the actual study, which examined niacin supplementation in roundworms and had nothing to say about bacon or humans. What was fascinating—and horrifying—about this particular example of social media "clickbait" was the way it had clearly manipulated a set of facts to garner attention. Science took a backseat to ad revenue.

I believe most people want to make good decisions about their health. Unfortunately, it can be hard to make good decisions when we are constantly being bombarded by misinformation in the media. Some people end up chasing fads, ultimately adopting the fatalistic attitude that if we can't know the truth, we might as well give up and enjoy ourselves.

Too often, this misdirection has to do with meat. In this essay, I'll show you two recent examples of how poorly conducted studies fooled lazy or ill-informed journalists into making animal products seem a whole lot healthier than they actually are. Let the reader and eater beware!

The first study was published in 2014 with the headline "Association of Dietary, Circulating, and Supplemental Fatty Acids with Coronary Risk." Soon after, *Time* magazine ran a cover story titled

"Eat Butter: Scientists labeled fat the enemy. Why they were wrong." The full-page image of an artfully curling pat of butter reinforced a tantalizing message: Advances in nutritional science had finally debunked the misguided (and depressing) notion that eating fat caused obesity and disease. And yet, the article produced no original research to back up this claim. In reality, it was a meta-analysis of seventy-two published studies that examined the associations between intake of different types of fat (polyunsaturated and saturated, principally) in different populations globally. The study's conclusion was that the "current evidence does not clearly support cardiovascular guidelines that encourage high consumption of polyunsaturated fatty acids and low consumption of total saturated fats."

THE EQUAL OF TWO EVILS IS NOT GOOD

From the beginning, it was clear *Time* magazine had mischaracterized the findings. The studies analyzed couldn't prove that vegetable oil is better than butter and lard. Put another way, imagine a study that compared cigarette smoking to tobacco chewing, and found that smoking wasn't much worse than chewing tobacco. A high school sophomore who wrote an essay called "Smoke Marlboros: Scientists labeled cigarettes the enemy. Why they were wrong," would receive a failing grade. At the same time, the study wasn't making a strong comparison. The only way to exonerate saturated fat was to compare it to unsaturated fat. A fairer and more meaningful analysis would have compared saturated fat to whole grains, or leafy greens, or potatoes. Anything else is a straw man argument.

LYING WITH STATISTICS

Have you seen the acronym GIGO? It stands for "garbage in, garbage out"—exactly what happened here. The majority of studies the authors chose to include employed statistical sleight of hand to erase the strong associations between saturated fat consumption and coronary disease. This sleight of hand was accomplished using a technique called statistical adjustment. This can be a fine and appropriate thing to do when you're comparing two groups that are different in meaningful ways. If you're comparing death rates from cancer in the USA and Botswana, for example, you have to account for the fact that the Botswana population is much younger, on average, than the US population. The goal of statistical adjustment is to remove numerical noise, but it can hide the truth if used to adjust for factors that directly influence the outcome.

And that's what the researchers in these studies did. They adjusted for calories consumed, blood pressure, body mass index (BMI), cholesterol, and fiber as well as intake of protein, carbohydrates, and vegetables. In other words, they were able to erase all differences between groups eating a lot and a little saturated fat by erasing all the ways saturated fat contributes to heart disease. Saturated fat contributes to heart disease by increasing calories consumed (meat and dairy are very calorically dense foods compared to fruits and vegetables), raising blood pressure by clogging arteries, increasing BMI, raising cholesterol, decreasing fiber intake by crowding out plant foods that contain fiber, increasing protein consumption (animal fat and protein go together in the diet), and decreasing consumption of carbohydrates and vegetables. Adjusting for these causal mechanisms is like adjusting for the velocity and weight of the bullet to prove that AK-47s aren't any deadlier than airsoft rifles.

CONVERTING ORANGES TO APPLES

The studies included in the meta-analysis were chosen specifically because they looked at groups eating more or less the same diet. And to make sure saturated fat got a clean bill of health, the author of this study evened out any remaining differences by using quintile transformations. For example, one study compared Japanese people who ate varying amounts of saturated fat, and another study looked at the same variation among people in Finland. In both cases, there was no correlation. Here's why: The Japanese people all ate small amounts of saturated fat. Even the biggest consumers in Japan ate much less than the lowest consumers in Finland. So when the two data sets were graphed and adjusted, they looked identical. But, if you compare Japanese to Finns, you get a totally different story. The Japanese rate of death from coronary disease was about 51 people per 100,000 people per year, while that of the Finns was 244, almost five times greater.

FAMILIAR TERRITORY

Similarly, a 2014 study titled "Effects of Low-Carbohydrate and Low-Fat Diets: A Randomized Trial" garnered serious headlines in the *New York Times*. The paper of record's lede on the topic was: "People who avoid carbohydrates and eat more fat, even saturated fat, lose more body fat and have fewer cardiovascular risks than people who follow the low-fat diet that health authorities have favored for decades, a major new study shows." Once the *Times* gave the study the stamp of legitimacy, other news outlets rushed to spread the good news that bacon and butter are better for us than chard and kale.

This study aims to be the gold standard of biomedical research, a randomized clinical trial. It took 148 people and randomly put them in a low-carb or a low-fat group and monitored their weight and a few cardiovascular risk factors (mostly their lipid panels). After a year, the low-carb group lost more weight and had better lipids than the low-fat group.

But should we all embrace high-protein, animal-based diets if we want to live healthier lives? Or is something else going on here? Let's peek under the hood of this study.

RETURN OF THE STRAW MAN

The biggest problem with this study is the definition of low-carb and low-fat. When the researchers define *low-fat* as "less than 30 percent of calories from fat," I have to invoke Mandy Patinkin's immortal line from *The Princess Bride*: "You keep using that word. I do not think it means what you think it means."

A truly low-fat diet would limit fat to 10 to 20 percent of calories, at the very most. Given that the standard American diet is about 35 percent fat, you can see that very little fat has to be eliminated to adhere to this "low-fat" label.

The low-carb group was instructed to consume less than 40 grams of carbohydrates daily. Given that no one has ever seen a carbohydrate, it's not surprising that they didn't achieve this goal. Actually, they exceeded it by over 200 percent, consuming an average 127 grams of carbs daily.

So we're drawing conclusions based on a comparison of a low-fat group that didn't eat low fat with a low-carb group that didn't eat low carb. And the *New York Times* wants us to pay attention to this?

We're left with a question: How come the supposed low-fat group didn't lose as much weight as the alleged low-carb group? Although the discussion within the published article claimed that "total energy intake was similar between groups," the reported data contradict this assessment. The low-fat group actually took in an average of 79 more calories per day than the low-carb group: 1,527 vs. 1,448.

Over the course of a year, that means the low-fat group consumed almost 29,000 more calories than the low-carb group. Given that it takes 3,500 calories to add a pound of fat, we can see that the low-fat group could be expected to gain 8.24 more pounds than the low-carb group simply based on consumption. Because the study reported that the difference in weight loss was only 7.7 pounds, this is explainable entirely based on the difference in calories. If *The New York Times* wishes to issue a retraction, may I suggest a better headline for this study: "Eating More Calories Increases Weight and Cardiovascular Risk Factors."

INOCULATE YOURSELF

This essay is far too short to give you all the tools necessary to recognize scientific mumbo jumbo when you see it. In general, though, if something appears too good to be true or contradicts prevailing wisdom, it's probably not worthy of breathless media coverage. Only after that study has been replicated a dozen times, especially by scientists skeptical of its conclusions, should it appear in our newspapers and our Facebook feeds.

BUILDING YOUR BODY WITH PLANTS

■ Robert Cheeke

Author of *Shred It!* and *Vegan Bodybuilding & Fitness*; two-time champion bodybuilder; founder/president of Vegan Bodybuilding & Fitness

In combination, the words *vegan bodybuilding* might seem like an oxymoron to many. And yet, they accurately describe my lifestyle over the past two decades. Since 1995, I have been a vegan athlete of one type or another, from runner to bodybuilder. During a stretch of eight years, I built my body from a 120-pound, newly vegan teenager, to a 195-pound champion bodybuilder. The entire time, I was battling against the belief—very common in mainstream fitness culture—that the massive consumption of animal products, especially animal protein, is synonymous with building muscle. This is simply not true; you can effectively build muscle on a reduced meat or plant-based diet. And I can prove it.

Though the overconsumption of animal products in athletic culture is still the norm, we are starting to see a shift in the awareness of the reduced meat lifestyle. Everyone from Olympic champions to weekend warriors are beginning to choose plants over animals when it comes to fueling their athletic pursuits. Our reasoning includes everything from preventing farm animal cruelty, to better health, to preserving the planet.

When evaluating nutritional choices as an athlete, the number of questions and uncertainties can seem endless. How much protein do we really need? Where should it come from? Are some forms of protein better than others? How many calories should I consume if I want to burn fat or build muscle? Should I avoid carbohydrates? However, if you grasp a few of the basic concepts, you'll be well equipped to attain your goals.

First, establish your basal metabolic rate (BMR). A search online will easily turn up a BMR calculator, which you can use to calculate your daily caloric expenditure based on your gender, age, height, and weight. Next, determine your caloric expenditure based on your average daily activity level using the Harris-Benedict equation, and combine the figures to get your true total caloric expenditure. Input your data using the "Harris-Benedict calculator" (also available online) to reveal your score. For example, at six feet tall, 185 pounds, thirty-five years of age, and male, my BMR shows that I burn 1,814 to 1,904 calories per day without doing any additional activities. When you factor in my exercise regimen, however, which includes weight training and plenty of cardio, I actually burn an additional 1,500 or so calories, making my total caloric expenditure ranging between 3,230 and 3,406 per day. This means, due to my active lifestyle, I need to eat 3,200 to 3,400 calories per day just to maintain weight. The numbers vary slightly from one Web site to another when using online calculators, but the range is close enough.

Not everybody is the same, of course—some people have more lean muscle mass, others may be affected by stress, hormones, thyroid function, and numerous other variables. What is most important to understand is that if your goal is to burn fat, you will need to reduce your caloric intake or increase your caloric expenditure to the point at which your expenditure exceeds your intake. The reverse is true for wanting to gain weight. In this scenario, if the excess calories consumed come from whole plant foods, combined with an effective weight-training program, muscle should be gained instead of fat. A traditional rule of thumb is that a caloric consumption deficit of 500 calories per day from your actual caloric expenditure will lead to about one pound of weight lost per week. This would total a 3,500-calorie deficit for the week, burning off a pound of fat. A pound of fat is roughly equivalent to 3,500 calories, so if consuming 500 fewer calories per day sounds too daunting, try reducing caloric intake by 250 calories per day and allow a couple of weeks for a pound of fat loss. As a warning: These numbers should be treated as more of a baseline rather than universally accurate. There are plenty of factors involved that can tweak the results somewhat, including the aforementioned lean body mass. Generally speaking, the more fat you have, the faster you will lose it on a calorie-deficit diet. If you have very little fat to lose, it will be a challenge to lose fat because our bodies naturally want to maintain a certain level of body fat for health, organ protection, and to protect against starvation.

Once you have established your true caloric expenditure and constructed a nutrition program with an appropriate caloric intake goal, you are ready to put the plan into motion. We now know that the human body requires only about 10 percent of its calories to come from protein. To build muscle while eating mostly plants, it's best to consume 70 percent of your calories via whole food complex carbohydrates and 15 percent of your calories from both fats and proteins. Plant foods contain significant amounts of vitamins, minerals, amino acids, fatty acids, fiber, water, phytonutrients, antioxidants, and other compounds that aid in healthy living. Plants are also free from dietary cholesterol. By eating a diverse diet of whole plant foods, you will obtain a nutrient-dense dietary plan to support your athletic endeavors.

As you can see, burning fat and building muscle do not require animal products. In fact, one could make the argument that a diet composed exclusively of plants might help accomplish fitness goals more efficiently, due to the nutrient density of whole plant foods. Not all foods are created equally, and some foods will provide a higher net nutritional return on investment than others. Just remember how many calories you need to consume—then throughout the day, you can tailor what you eat to reach your targets. When combined with a consistent exercise program, this type of diet provides the recipe for success.

For the exercise portion of your new lifestyle, remember that consistency, accountability, and transparency are very important. Document your workouts so you have an accurate record of your work. If weight training is part of your program, try to use free-weight dumbbells and barbells for compound, multijoint movements that stimulate muscle growth. Whether weight training, endurance, or a team sport is your focus, provide ample time to warm up, stretch, recover, and prevent injuries from overuse so you can keep your routine on track.

Ultimately, there is simply no need to consume animal products to burn fat, build muscle, or attain other fitness goals. Train hard, eat well, and learn and understand the science behind your pursuit— and enjoy your fitness journey.

HUMAN HEALTH AND THE MYTHOLOGY OF MEAT

■ David L. Katz

Director, Yale University Prevention Research Center; president, American College of Lifestyle Medicine; founder, the Truth Health Coalition

We *Homo sapiens* are constitutionally omnivorous, and have been since before *sapiens* was appended to the family name. That means we have choices.

While processed meat has been robustly, if not definitively, associated with adverse health outcomes, the same is not true of, say, antelope or venison or wild salmon. The distinction is worth emphasizing: Much of the meat that most people eat in the modern context is potentially hazardous to health, associated with inflammation, dyslipidemia, atherosclerosis, and increases in chronic disease risk.

But such meats as those are nearly as far from the versions truly native to the *Homo sapiens* experience as is diet soda relative to water. Meat, per se, is surely not toxic to human health.

Why? Because there is nothing intrinsically toxic about any given potential food. What determines toxicity is not so much the food, as the feeder, or better yet, the interaction between the two and the environmental context. Eucalyptus leaves are considerably toxic to cats, dogs, and horses, yet clearly rather the contrary for koala bears. If fish accumulate toxins because we have adulterated our oceans, the fault lies not with the fish but our environmental abuses. Toxicity is defined by adaptation and physiology. Famously, one man's meat is another man's poison, and that much more so when comparing across species.

Exactly the same is true of essential nutrients or foods. The limits of biological adaptation, and any given species' expression of them, define what is essential. Universal assertions about necessary sustenance suffer the same liabilities as such declarations about toxicity.

The ardent advocates of our Stone Age hunting, or at least the modern mythology built around it, often go so far as to contend that eating meat is essential for optimal health. One argument is that meat eating was a factor in the marked increase in the size of our brains and is now vital to feed those large brains. Another argument is that meat and its high-quality protein are essential to optimize the form and function of our own muscles.

Both contentions are, in a word, baloney. Just consider gorillas, who build their massive muscle from a diet that is 97 percent vegetarian, the small remainder coming from termites and caterpillars. Or for that matter, consider a horse, such as the magnificent, Triple Crown–winning American Pharaoh: a mountain of sleek muscle built entirely from plants. Meat is not required to build muscle. Rather, animal muscle can be built from any fuel that kind of animal is adapted to burn. We *Homo sapiens* are, as noted, adapted to burn both plant and animal food.

As for brains, there are predatory animals with far smaller brains (or, more important, brain size to body size ratio, which is the defining metric of species intelligence) than ours, and others with larger brains; and the same is true of plant eaters. The animals with intelligence most approximating our own are vegetarians, or nearly so.

The argument that our big brains arose in the context of eating meat and therefore we must eat meat now is no more valid than the argument that our big brains arose in the context of dodging large predators and hitting rival clan members over the head with cudgels, so we should release lions, tigers, and bears into every suburb and hit one another over the head routinely. Environmental associations do not cause-and-effect requirement make.

We are neither carnivores nor herbivores. We are constitutional omnivores. There are specific aspects of our physiology particular to meat consumption, and perhaps even the consumption of cooked meat per se. There are adaptations even since the advent of civilization that are particular to dairy consumption. Valid arguments over the place of dietary meat and dairy in human health are far more challenging and nuanced than the opposing clamors would suggest and might well come down to: What meat and which kind of dairy?

Meat is not intrinsically toxic to our natively omnivorous species. Claims that it is are at odds with the elegant logic of evolution by natural selection; the two are unavoidably in conflict. But even so, we may reasonably decide that any dietary choice that places on the menu the perpetration of cruelty upon our fellow species is toxic. We may reasonably decide that any dietary choice unsustainable by more than 7 billion *Homo sapiens* is now, in that context, toxic. We may reasonably conclude that accelerating the depletion of aquifers is toxic. These ancillary considerations about meat are worth chewing. I cannot improve on a recent headline in IFL-Science!: "Meat Is a Complex Health Issue but a Simple Climate One." Amen.

Meat is not essential for *Homo sapiens* either. There are vegans among the world's most elite athletes. There are vegetarians among the world's great intellectuals. But the most ardent vegetarians might constructively concede that we have no true evidence that an optimal diet of only plants (vegan) is better for human health than an optimal diet of mostly plants (Mediterranean).

Perhaps the best resolution of the matter, and one entirely concordant with the reducetarian principle, is derived neither from fantasies about the Stone Age nor the canonization of cauliflower but from the real-world experience of entire populations over generations. To date, all of the Blue Zone populations discovered, recognized for exceptional longevity and vitality, practice variations on the same basic dietary theme: wholesome foods, mostly plants, in sensible combinations.

We *Homo sapiens* are neither constitutionally carnivorous, like cheetahs, nor constitutionally herbivorous, like the impalas they pursue. We are constitutionally omnivorous, and that means we have choices to make. We have ample information and robust reasons to make sensible choices—based on our own health, the treatment of our fellow species, the sustainability of resources, and the fate of our planet.

There can be a place for meat in human diets, assuming the meat is wholesome, from animals fed their native diets, and spared incarceration or abuse. But aggregate evidence regarding both human health and the health of the planet indicates clearly: that place should be small.

MEATLESS MONDAY: ONE DAY A WEEK, CUT OUT MEAT

■ Sid Lerner

Founder of the Meatless Monday movement

People often ask me about Meatless Monday—why meat, why Monday. For years we've known that eating too much meat isn't healthy, and research shows us that eating more than we should is directly linked to obesity, heart disease, diabetes, and cancer. These days it's not genes or germs killing us; it's what we're eating that's making us sick. And then there's the environmental cost: raising, processing, and shipping meat generates massive amounts of pollution and greenhouse gases. We all know we should be eating less meat, but for years it has stayed at the center of the plate. I started Meatless Monday twelve years ago to help people get healthier by giving up meat just once a week.

I'd been in the ad business for years and thought: Why not sell health instead of products? Back then, doctors were telling us to cut meat intake by 15 percent. I did the math, and that came out to one day in seven, three meals out of twenty-one. Cut the meat one day a week, and you wouldn't have to look at every plate and ask how to get rid of 15 percent of the meat. Just three meals, one day a week, don't eat meat. It was simple and easy to remember.

Why'd I pick Monday? Back when I was a boy scout there was a campaign called Meatless Monday to help conserve food for the troops in World War II. Meatless Monday was a tidy and timely way to package the healthy idea; doable and understandable, those two words said it all.

The movement started off slowly, but that reasonable, plausible phrase has made a real impact. Brands like Boca Burger used it to promote healthy eating to consumers. In 2009, Baltimore City Public Schools began offering Meatless Monday lunches to students; hundreds of schools have jumped on the bandwagon since then.

Celebrities like Oprah and Michael Pollan have gotten involved, and Chef Mario Batali brought the movement to his restaurants with special Meatless Monday dishes.

Sir Paul McCartney helped us take Meatless Monday global in 2009 by launching Meat Free Monday in the UK. Now nearly forty countries around the world are a part of the movement. Here in the United States, whole cities have adopted Meatless Monday. Many, including Cleveland, Los Angeles, Philadelphia, San Francisco, and Washington, D.C., have passed Meatless Monday resolutions encouraging residents and businesses to join in.

Meatless Monday helps get the idea into the mind before getting it into the body. Every seven days you have a chance to start and maintain new good habits or break old bad ones. Research shows that we're more interested in health on Monday than on any other day of the week. People start diets, begin exercise routines, quit smoking, and search for health information on the Internet more on Mondays. And surveys show that if you're going to make a healthy change that sticks, Monday is the best day of the week to start.

With diet-related diseases on the rise and communication easier than ever before, now is a critical time to talk about healthy eating. I founded Meatless Monday because when I looked around twelve years ago, I didn't see anyone getting public health information out to the people who needed to hear it. At Meatless Monday, we use marketing techniques to help bring public health to the public.

You don't have to change everything to get healthier. This campaign doesn't tell you to become a vegetarian or expect you to give up your favorite foods. Just take one day a week and get the beef and chicken off your buns and give Meatless Monday a try.

IT'S TIME TO EAT!

▌ Lindsay Nixon

Author of the best-selling *The Happy Herbivore* cookbook
series and CEO of Meal Mentor

There are two main things to keep in mind when you are thinking about reducing your meat consumption (even if you don't plan to commit 100 percent, 100 percent of the time). First, take the process one meal at a time. Don't worry about what's going to happen at Thanksgiving in a few months or what you'll do at a cousin's wedding next year. Focus on your next meal and making it work.

Second, don't try to go from 0 to 180 right out of the gate. It's not an easy change, and just like trying anything for the first time, there's bound to be a massive learning curve. If you decided to train for a marathon today, you wouldn't expect to lace up your sneakers and go run 20 miles on your first day. You'd start with 5 miles or maybe even 1 mile. You'd work your way up, mile by mile, week after week, until you were prepared to run the full 26.2 miles. Treat diet and lifestyle changes the same way. Start with small things you can maintain. Be realistic or you won't last a week, no matter how strong your intentions.

Know, too, that you are already busy and overstretched, so adding more to your to do list is probably not a good idea. Instead of adding on, subtract. For example, it's a lot easier to *stop* drinking wine or eating beef than it is to suddenly *start* going to the gym five times a week at 6:00 A.M.

I find it can be helpful to create two new rules for yourself right at the start. Maybe you want your rules to be "I don't eat chicken" or "I don't eat fish." Be specific and affirmative—no gray areas or "I will trys" or exceptions. Draw that line in the sand and make sure you know exactly where you stand. And then you don't cross it. This practice also means you won't have to worry about mustering up enough willpower—you can't talk yourself into or out of something if the decision's already been made.

When it comes time to actually start cooking, why not begin by tweaking your favorite meals in easy ways. This way, the food will still be familiar, even if it is more plant based. For example, chickpeas and white mushrooms make a great replacement for chicken in recipes. You can also substitute black beans, bulgur wheat, quinoa, brown mushrooms (chopped) and textured vegetable protein (TVP) for ground beef. Portobellos (whole or in strips) make for a great steak substitute!

There's also no shortage of commercial vegan meat replacements (Field Roast and Gardein are popular brands), not to mention the more basic, blank canvas options like tofu, tempeh, and seitan. (Keep in mind that while these substitutes are easy and often helpful during a dietary transition, for optimal health you will want to focus on whole foods in the long term.) When I first stopped eating meat, I realized I actually cared more about the sauces than the meat they were served with—meat was just the vehicle to get the sauce in my mouth. The good news is, you can still enjoy ketchup, barbecue sauce, marinara, and all of our favorite sauces—and feel healthy while doing it.

Spices and herbs can also provide the flavors you know and love without your actually eating any animal-based ingredients. For example, kelp (a sea vegetable) lends a fabulous fishy taste to seafood-like dishes. I also find liquid smoke, mixed with a touch of maple syrup, recreates a ham flavor quite well, while black salt adds an eggy aspect and rubbed sage can create a lovely sausage essence. Part of the fun (yes fun!) of developing a new diet is exploring new flavors, cuisines, and spice combinations. I eat a much wider variety of foods now than I ever did previously, and often find myself seeking out new food experiences or ingredients I've never tried before.

It's likely that you'll also notice your palate, tastes, and cravings change. Once a glutton for cupcakes, I now think they're much too sweet and would much prefer a crisp, fresh apple or a really juicy mango instead. On that note, have a little patience as your tastes acclimate to a new, healthful diet. Processed foods (and restaurant foods) are loaded with salt, sugar, and oil—a super addictive combination.

The more sugar, salt, and oil you eat, the more you crave it. But these "foods" have another adverse effect: They rob you of experiencing true flavor. Oil coats your tongue like a glove while salt and sugar overstimulate and damage your taste receptors. Fortunately, taste buds heal and become sensitive again. Be patient—the process may take a few weeks, during which time food may seem extremely bland. But I promise the wait is worth it. You won't believe what you've been missing!

Finally, whenever you start to feel limited or like you're missing out, focus on all the foods you *can* enjoy, not the one you chose to pass up. (Notice I didn't say the foods you "can't have"—because you can have them if you want, you've simply chosen not to.) This is also a strategy used by people with food allergies. Anytime I start to feel frustrated by my special dietary needs, I start thinking instead about all the things I *can* have. Why stare at a closed door when you could be gazing out a window? Remember, there was a good reason you chose to make these changes. At the end of the day, my food is fuel—it's what I need to have fun, not the fun itself. You don't go to weddings and birthdays for the food, you go for the experiences and the memories. And with that, it's time to eat!

ANTIBIOTIC RESISTANCE AT THE MEAT COUNTER

Lance B. Price

Director, Antibiotic Resistance Action Center (ARAC), Milken Institute School of Public Health, George Washington University

As a public health researcher, I can tell you that there are lots of reasons you should decrease the amount of meat you eat. But as a microbiologist, the part of meat consumption that concerns me the most is our exposure to disease-causing bacteria resistant to antibiotics. Also known as superbugs, this type of scary bacteria is rampant in today's food supply.

Each year in the United States, about 2 million people are infected with superbugs and at least 23,000 die. *Salmonella* and *Campylobacter*—two bacteria that are frequently transmitted via contaminated meat and poultry—cause 410,000 of these antibiotic-resistant infections.[1] And now we're learning that meat can carry other drug-resistant pathogens as well. For example, my colleagues and I recently discovered that *Klebsiella pneumoniae* frequently contaminates the pork, chicken, and turkey products sold in grocery stores. This nasty bug can cause antibiotic-resistant urinary tract infections, liver abscesses, and bloodstream infections.

I have dedicated my career to stopping the spread of superbugs, and central to this goal is ending the overuse and misuse of antibiotics in food-animal production. Science tells us that bacteria move about freely in the environment and some superbugs flow seamlessly between people and animals. Studies dating back to the 1960s have shown repeatedly how antibiotic use in food-animal production helps breed superbugs that eventually end up in our food, air and water.

Groups such as the World Health Organization (WHO) and the U.S. Centers for Disease Control and Prevention (CDC) have said that if we don't significantly reduce antibiotic use in all settings— human, animal, and agriculture—we will soon be living in a post-antibiotic world. Transplants and cancer treatments will no longer be possible, surgery and childbirth could have deadly consequences for tens of millions of people, and even a superficial cut could kill. Antibiotics are the cornerstones of modern medicine, but if we don't find ways to protect the drugs from needless overuse, their days of protecting us from deadly bacteria will come to an end.

One of the things I find most alarming is the amount of antibiotics sold for use in chickens, turkeys, cattle, and pigs here in the United States. The most recent data from the U.S. Food and Drug Administration shows that 32.6 million pounds of antibiotics were sold for use in food animals in 2013. Compare that against the most recent data for humans—7.7 million pounds of antibiotics sold to treat people in 2011.[2] When fed to animals, most of these drugs are used to promote rapid growth or to keep animals from getting sick due to their often unsanitary and overcrowded living conditions. Animals destined for the dinner table consume about four times the amount of antibiotics prescribed by the medical system. Yet, most of the efforts to curb antibiotic use have focused on the human side.

Antibiotic resistance is a serious global threat to public health. Everyone has a role to play in combating it, including food-animal producers, the pharmaceutical industry, and policymakers. If you do buy meat, be careful when handling raw meat in the store and when you get it home. In addition, there are numerous food safety practices that you can adhere to that should lessen your exposure to bacteria on raw meat. These include washing your hands and kitchen surfaces often, refraining from washing raw meat (as that tends to spread bacteria), using separate cutting boards for meat and produce, cooking meat at its proper temperature and storing it properly. The CDC Web site also has excellent information on the subject for meat consumers.

Of course, meat eaters are not the only people who should be concerned about antibiotic resistance; antibiotic resistance is everyone's problem. Bacteria can be transported from place to place via human contact, water, wind, or air. When this happens, resistance spreads through communities, hospitals, and farms. Drug-resistant bacteria in fertilizer or water used on food crops can even come home in your grocery bag. Moreover, as I noted earlier, antibiotic resistance is causing antibiotics to lose their effectiveness. Ultimately, everyone has a role to play in combating antibiotic resistance, including consumers who can vote with their wallets to support companies that use antibiotics responsibly.

WISDOM FROM MARGARET MEAD

■ Bee Wilson

Author of *First Bite: How We Learn to Eat* and *Consider the Fork: A History of How We Cook and Eat*

Like children, most of us eat what we like and we like what we know. One thing about food that seems to be near-universally popular is having "more" of it. We prefer our portions to be generous, not stingy. The word *more* suggests largesse and second helpings. It means bottomless coffee—or a takeout cup so large you can't see the bottom of it—and not worrying where the next meal will come from. Any project encouraging us to eat less of something—in this case, meat—will struggle to find many followers unless it can somehow recast less as "more."

During World War II, the anthropologist Margaret Mead was asked by the National Research Council to look into how American civilians might be persuaded to change their food habits. How could the constraints of rationing be accepted? In particular, Mead focused on how Americans could be encouraged to cope with an "undersupply" of meat. There were various possible approaches, Mead noted. The most obvious approach was negative: The government could emphasize "simple lack of meat, or simple need to eat substitutes if we are to live." But such gloomy messages, in Mead's view, had "pitfalls." Emphasizing the lack of meat could create a mind-set of deprivation and anger ("Are we to go back to the terrible days of the Depression?"). When people feel deprived, they yearn for the halcyon state when they can splurge once again. Meat becomes more, not less desirable. As Mead commented, such a mind-set probably partly explains why sugar consumption rocketed after World War I.

A more promising approach, Mead felt, was to emphasize the scientific benefits of eating less meat. If people could be told that eating alternative proteins was based on "the best available nutritional science," then reduced amounts of meat might actually seem a positive choice. Instead of aching for the time when meat would be plentiful again, people could use the war as "an opportunity to break away" from a "poorly balanced diet." Eating less meat during the war could be a "rehearsal" for a new way of life in times of peace.

We, clearly, are living through very different times from the wartime generation (though the current food scarcity in Venezuela is a reminder that we cannot rely on ingredients being plentiful forever). In the affluent West, meat eaters can choose from overflowing counters of roasts, sausages, steaks, and ribs.

Those with money to buy it are free to eat all the meat they like, and they do like. Because of mass production, it doesn't even cost as much as it did a few decades ago. "During the war," recalled the British food writer Marguerite Patten, "chickens were rarely seen in butchers' shops." Not anymore.

Yet the questions that Mead was grappling with about how to adjust a meat habit remain as important as ever. Campaigners and governments can persuade large numbers of people to cut down on the meat they consume each week only by addressing the psychology of eating less. How can we make a pizza without pepperoni seem more desirable than a pizza with pepperoni?

When you utter the phrase *meat free* to meat eaters, you are sending a signal that they are missing out on something. A meatless meal sounds less than a carnivorous meal. It is defining itself by what it is not. This is the potential trouble with all of those well-meaning meat-free initiatives such as Meat Free Monday. Thousands of people have a Monday night dinner of black bean chili sin carne, feel virtuous for abstaining from meat, and then return with relief to short ribs and hamburgers for the rest of the week.

If we want to make more radical cuts to our meat habit, we need to flip our mind-set around. Given that we mostly eat what we like, lasting change is most likely to come from learning new preferences. Scientists have known for decades that the main way that anyone—adult or child—learns to like new foods is simply by trying them, multiple times, in a positive environment. In 1968, psychologist Robert Zajonc coined the term *mere exposure* to describe this effect, which has since been confirmed across cultures. The work of biologists Gary Beauchamp and Julie Mennella has confirmed that a baby born to a mother who drinks a lot of carrot juice will learn to love the flavor of carrots.

The problem with our excessive meat habit—in common with our sugar habit and many other damaging behaviors—is that it is self-reinforcing. Every time we celebrate with barbecue or cheer ourselves up with a juicy steak or pick a ham sandwich as our default lunch, we are conditioning ourselves to think that life with less meat would somehow be pinched and dull or weird and uncomfortable.

We could, however, adopt Margaret Mead's approach and try to see a vegetable-centric diet as something delicious and superior, rather than a deprivation. As an individual, it is possible to reach the point at which a meal of falafel and hummus with crunchy pickled carrots and soft roasted eggplant seems like more of a treat than a greasy meatball sub. This change won't happen straight away. As with teaching a child to eat, it will likely take multiple exposures before you develop a taste for bitter greens or realize that the texture of tofu—so spongy and sinister at first—can be comforting. Food habits permanently alter only when dislikes turn to likes.

If we seriously want to limit meat eating, we should focus on making the meatless meal seem like the better, rather than the lesser, option. It is not a case of making do with less but of realizing that, actually, everything doesn't taste better with bacon. Given the ongoing kale obsession, there are signs that a significant minority of eaters is already starting to respond to food in this way. Chefs such as Yotam Ottolenghi have helped to make such dishes as chickpea sauté or sweet potato cakes more desirable than meat. When you are in the habit of cooking these new-wave vegetable recipes—heady with herbs and tahini—there is no deprivation. The title of one of Ottolenghi's books is *Plenty*. The great question remains what it would take for the population at large to feel that a life with less meat can still be plenty.

FARM TO SCHOOL AND SALAD BARS: GETTING KIDS EATING MORE FRUIT AND VEGGIES!

■ Ann Cooper

Co-author of *Lunch Lessons: Changing the Way We Feed Our Children*

We all know that we need to eat more fruits and veggies, and nowhere is that more important than in schools. If we want our children to live long, healthy lives, then we need to teach them that at least 50 percent of their trays need to be filled with plant-based foods. Fresh fruit, fresh vegetables, whole grains and plant-based proteins must become part of our school meals, and most important they need to be eaten by the kids. If we expect to change our children's relationship to food and hope to get them to eat healthier, then the food they eat in schools and the education that surrounds it is of the utmost import. In this vein, there are a number of impactful tools that we can use, including farm to school programs, school gardens, and salad bars.

The U.S. Department of Agriculture (USDA) recognizes the national farm to school movement as consisting of efforts to bring local or regionally produced foods into the school cafeteria while introducing students to hands-on classroom learning activities that connect them to their food. This movement encompasses a wide range of initiatives, such as school gardening; farm visits; the integration of agriculture, food production and preparation; and nutrition-related education into the current standards-based curriculum.

"An investment in the health of America's students through farm-to-school activities is also an investment in the health of local economies," says Agriculture Secretary Tom Vilsack. "We know that when students have experiences such as tending a school garden or visiting a farm, they'll be more likely to make healthy choices in the cafeteria. We also know that when schools invest their food dollars in their local communities, all of agriculture benefits, including local farmers, ranchers, fishermen, food processors and manufacturers."

Engaging kids at the farm level is also a great learning tool. Farm to school relationships can help reinforce where their food comes from. Farms are starting to show up even within the city limits of large cities (for example, Detroit and Denver) as local organizations address the issue of food access in the United States. Students' experiences at farmers' markets or student-run farmers' markets is another excellent option for building relationships between kids and food; what does a food look like in the field, what do the seeds look like, how does it taste raw or cooked?

In a survey conducted in the 2011–2012 academic year, the USDA found that more than 43 percent of all U.S. school districts were engaged in some sort of farm to school programming. Here are some examples of these initiatives:

- Procuring local food
- Building school gardens
- Hosting culinary classes and cook-off events using local produce
- Visiting local farms
- Designing curriculum tie-ins with agriculture and nutrition
- Creating new farmers' markets at local schools
- Developing districtwide planting and harvesting events
- Fruit and vegetable tastings

The desired outcome from these educational endeavors is that students not only eat more plant-based foods in school but also take their education and palates home, where they begin to positively impact family meals. One of the best companion pieces to farm to school programming is salad bars.

Research shows that incorporating salad bars into school lunches increases children's consumption of fresh fruits and vegetables. Salad bars profoundly shift the typical school lunch by offering students not only variety but also choice. Schools with salad bars offer a wider variety of vegetables and fruits than other schools. Through repeat exposure, encouragement to try unfamiliar foods, and education, children respond by trying new items, incorporating greater variety into their diets, and eating more fruits and vegetables each day. As a result of these early, positive experiences, students develop palates for a lifetime of healthy eating.

To maximize these benefits, the White House Task Force on Childhood Obesity, in their May 2010 Report to the president, endorses the use of salad bars in schools and upgrading cafeteria equipment to provide healthy meals for kids. The Healthy Hunger-Free Kids Act of 2010 and the resulting new school meal guidelines that went into effect in 2012 support increasing vegetable and fruit consumption by changing the school lunch requirements to 6.25 to 10 servings of fruits and vegetables weekly. The USDA encourages the use of salad bars in school meal programs, stating, "Salad bars continue to be a great option for meeting the meal pattern requirements."

The Let's Move Salad Bars to Schools Initiative launched in 2010. As of 2014, the initiative—through donations totaling more than $10 million—has donated more than 4,100 salad bars across the country and brought fresh vegetable and fruits choices to over 2 million students in participating schools. Today, the salad bar is a proven, accessible tool to (1) improve school meals in an immediate way and (2) comply with the various vegetable subgroups under the New Meal Pattern Requirements and Nutrition Standards for the USDA's National School Lunch and School Breakfast Programs. Many more school districts are now implementing salad bars as a core part of their food service operations.

Food education is important and can contribute to a healthy learning environment and academic success. Creating choices at the salad bar opens up a whole new world of experiences for students. Encouraging them to try new foods is one of the most important tasks given to both the food service and education teams. Identifying foods, tasting new foods, creating composed salads that provide blended tastes—these are all very important lessons that can help students develop healthy eating habits that support classroom success.

PLANET

Out of all those millions and millions of planets floating around there in space, this is our planet, this is our little one, so we just got to be aware of it and take care of it.
—PAUL McCARTNEY

ROLL YOUR OWN: WEEKDAY VEGETARIAN

■ Graham Hill

Founder of LifeEdited.com and TreeHugger.com

Several years ago, I asked myself a question: "Knowing what I know, why am I not a vegetarian?" I consider myself a green guy. I grew up with hippie parents in a log cabin. I started a site called TreeHugger.com, devoted to sustainability, design, food, culture, transportation, energy, fashion, politics, health, and other environmental issues. I knew that the billions of animals we eat are raised in packed-to-the-gills, feces-filled factory farms. I knew meat production has a bigger carbon footprint than all transportation forms combined: cars, trains, planes, buses, and boats . . . all of it! And I knew eating a mere hamburger a day could increase my risk of premature death by a third and that beef production uses 100 times more water than vegetable production does. Yet there I was, twiddling my thumbs, chomping on my burger like everything was cool.

I know vegetarianism is better for the planet, our health, and animals—but in our carnivorous culture, it can be hard to make the change. Though we as a society are eating less meat than we did a decade ago, we still eat twice as much as we did in the 1950s. What was once a meal's special little side treat has become its star attraction.

So why was I stalling? I think it was because I had created a binary solution: You're either a meat eater or you're a vegetarian. I wasn't sure if I was ready to make the full plunge. Even though there are many delicious plant-based meals, my common sense and good intentions often conflicted with my taste buds. With this binary solution, my timetable for going veg was always the same: I'll do it later. It is not surprising that later never came.

As time passed, I wondered if there might be a third solution—something between never eating meat and eating it all the time?

After all, if everyone reduced their meat consumption by half, it would be like half of us were vegetarians. That was when I came up with weekday vegetarianism. The name says it all: I wouldn't eat anything that had a face on it Monday through Friday. On the weekend, the choice was mine. It's simple and structured, so it is easy to remember, and it's flexible enough that I could break it here and there without feeling restricted. After all, cutting out meat five days a week is equivalent to cutting 70 percent of my overall intake. This decrease results in a smaller carbon footprint; a longer, healthier life; a reduction in the suffering of animals; and probably more money in my wallet. If you're looking to reduce your meat consumption, I can't recommend weekday vegetarianism enough.

But if weekday vegetarianism doesn't mesh with your lifestyle, that's all right too. It's just one strategy among many for eating less meat and for being a reducetarian. Two other possible variations are (1) The Vampire: Eats meat only after the sun has set and (2) The Deck o' Cards: Eats meat no bigger than a deck of cards.

The point is to do what works for you. The important thing is to make consistent progress toward your objective of curbing meat consumption. Every little reduction helps improve both personal and planetary health. My current venture, LifeEdited.com, is about designing happier, greener lives using less space and stuff than the status quo would have us believe is necessary. But not everyone is ready to give up his or her 4,000-square-foot home for a 200-square-foot micro apartment. Maybe they start with reducing their home size to 3,000 square feet. Progress is the point. That said, the more you reduce—whether it's meat or housing size—the more you help.

In this process, it's important to be compassionate with ourselves. We must understand our limitations and obstacles. Sometimes we are going to lack the fortitude to live up to our ideals. No undertaking is perfect. Often, reaching an objective such as cutting out or significantly reducing meat consumption is an incremental process, fraught with missteps and compromises. Sure, absolute dedication is a laudable quality, but you don't need to be unbending to make progress. For example, special occasions like traveling abroad or staying with friends or family might call for more permissiveness—you want to taste the local cuisine that is cooked with pork or you want to eat Thanksgiving turkey on Thanksgiving (a weekday). Don't stress out. Even if you take a short break from eating less meat, you can always return to some tasty, heart-and-earth-friendly veggie dishes. Every bit helps. Keep your goals realistic, keep moving forward and you will find it just gets easier and easier to eat less meat.

MEAT IS PRECIOUS

▌ Bill McKibben

Author, educator, environmentalist, and co-founder of 350.org

Helping build the grassroots climate movement has meant a lot of travel. In the last few years I've journeyed to all seven continents, often meeting with people who exist at the very bottom of the economic heap, the ones who have done the least to cause environmental trouble and yet feel its effects most harshly. Along the way, I learned something surprising: An awful lot of these people are getting the opportunity to eat meat for the first time in their lives, and they're enjoying it. I remember talking to an old man in a slum on the edge of Beijing, asking him why he'd left his village to come to the smoky city. "In my village we had no alcohol, and we had no meat," he said. And that was that.

Meanwhile, in the developed world, I've met lots of people who believe we should all become vegans immediately in order to save the planet. Some of them are kind about it, and some (often the newly converted), are not. I have no doubts about their zeal, but I do worry about their effectiveness. This is a problem because their basic message is extremely important: reducing factory farming of animals would help a lot in the fight against global warming.

That's why reducetarianism interests me so much. Its message strikes me as far more effective than moralizing, especially if the end goal is to convince more people to reduce their meat consumption. The reducetarianism movement meets most people on our planet more or less at their level—they enjoy the taste of meat and yet also worry about our planet's future. Reducetarianism also honors the cuisines of the developing world, places where meat has long been used as a condiment and a flavoring instead of the Great Honking Steak technique more common in the United States.

To lay it out mathematically, if you could convert 5 percent of the population to veganism, that would be a very good thing. It would also be quite difficult—so far, about 1 million Americans, or 0.5 percent, have been convinced to take that step. But in carbon terms, it would be far more useful to convince one third or one half of Americans to cut their meat consumption by a third or a half. And that strikes me as a far more achievable organizing task. When you lay it out for them, most people can understand the health benefits and cost savings of reduced meat consumption. Some might even be excited for the culinary possibilities. On the other hand, a movement that is perceived as compromising won't give advocates quite the same feeling of self-righteousness, which is either a good thing or a bad thing depending on your preference.

It's been a long time since I've cooked a hamburger. But I do eat one on occasion, primarily in places where someone has killed the fatted calf because guests from the outside world have arrived. To refuse in such situations always seems churlish, not to mention counterproductive. Having spent the carbon to travel somewhere as an organizer, the last thing I want to do is offend my hosts. Rather, I'd like to honor their gift, and use it as an opportunity to suggest that meat is precious and something to be used sparingly. I'm grateful to the reducetarians for making this last goal easier—and for helping point out some routes that should ultimately take us where we all want to go.

LESS MEAT TAKES A BITE OUT OF GLOBAL HUNGER

■ Dawn Moncrief

Founding director of A Well Fed World

Good news—reducing personal meat consumption has been proven to have even farther-reaching benefits than previously anticipated. In addition to the oft-cited health, environmental, and animal protection improvements, reducing meat consumption also positively impacts global hunger concerns and global food security more generally.

The livestock industry undermines hunger alleviation efforts in many ways, from climate change to pollution to energy consumption. This essay, however, is going to specifically focus on the livestock industry's crop use inefficiencies. Put simply, farmed animals consume much more food than they produce. A recent report calculates that 36 percent of the world's crops are used as animal feed, yet only 12 percent of that total winds up contributing to the human diet as animal-sourced foods.[1]

The stark caloric inefficiency that occurs when farms convert staple crops (wheat, corn, soy, etc.) into meat is reflected clearly in feed conversion ratios (FCRs). Feed conversion ratios refer to the amount of animal feed/crops needed to produce a unit of live weight gain or unit of edible meat. For example, a 10:1 ratio means that ten pounds of food must be consumed by an animal to produce one pound of weight gain (live weight FCRs) or one pound of ready-to-purchase meat (edible meat FCRs). Feed conversion ratios are important, but they can be confusing. As a general rule of thumb, calculation details should be included whenever possible, as FCRs vary greatly depending on species/breed, rearing/processing methods, presenter bias, and a multitude of other factors.

Despite FCR variability, some generalizations and observations can be made. For instance, to promote animal agriculture as efficient, the livestock industry often uses the more conservative live weight FCRs, which downplay the immense crop consumption of animals raised for food. It's more accurate to consider the amount of crops needed to produce a unit of edible meat (after bones, blood, excess fat, and other nonedible parts are removed). Edible meat FCRs are usually between two and three times higher (more inefficient) than live weight FCRs.

At the low end, the poultry industry often boasts a 2:1 live weight FCR, meaning that chickens eat about two pounds of feed for every one pound of weight gained. Of course, if 50 percent of food was being wasted by a restaurant, it would be cause for great concern. Yet when 50 percent of crops are lost in the conversion to poultry meat, livestock lobbyists celebrate. Indeed, poultry is often hailed as the most efficient land-based livestock, yet after deboning, fluid draining, and other processing, our caloric investment yields low returns. For larger animals, the inefficiencies run much higher. According to scientist and policy analyst Vaclav Smil, the edible meat FCR for pigs is more than 9:1, while the ratio jumps to 25:1 for cows.[2] By this calculation, grain-fed cattle require roughly twenty-five pounds of staple crops to produce just one pound of beef.

With over 70 billion land animals slaughtered annually, livestock's immense role in resource depletion as well as its lack of sustainability is cause for serious concern. In addition to these problems, high levels of animal-sourced food consumption can lead to food price increases. Not to overstate the causal relationship—factors such as speculation, protectionism, and subsidies remain influential—but generally speaking, high demand for animal feed crops puts upward pressure on food prices. Higher prices in turn often lead to decreased purchasing power, especially for the world's urban poor, who already spend a large percentage of their income on food. To the degree that supply can readily keep pace with demand, food prices tend to be more stable. However, with expanding population, increasingly scarce natural resources and intensifying climate disruptions, food supply is likely to tighten relative to demand if meat consumption remains unchecked.

Anyone concerned about the negative consequences of food waste and/or biofuel use should be even more concerned about the livestock industry. Many of its problems related to crop use/waste are far greater, and the environmental consequences potentially more catastrophic. Indeed, given the crop-intensive and resource-intensive nature of animal agriculture, unnecessary meat consumption could be seen as a wasteful form of overconsumption. Similarly, wasted meat can be considered a "multiplier of waste," further compounded by meat's highly perishable nature. On the upside, reducing or eliminating meat and other animal-sourced foods can be considered a form of food and resource conservation. The greater the reduction, the higher the reward.

While the United States is one of the world's highest ranking per capita consumers of meat, recent years have seen a decline in aggregate national consumption despite increases in population. Globally, however, meat consumption is rising dramatically. In emerging economies—where growth is greatest—meat is often considered a "prestige food," and consumption is fueled in part by a desire to emulate wealthier countries. Reduced meat consumption among the world's higher-income consumers therefore provides a vital counternarrative, setting a better example and improving our credibility on hunger and environmental issues.

Thus, in addition to tangible improvements in the global food system, meat reduction also positively impacts cultural norms and policymaking. Similar gains can be achieved by reinforcing meat reductionist trends at the national level. Meat reducers bolster the popularity of plant-based foods and meat alternatives. This spurs greater investment and product development in plant-based foods, making reduced meat consumption more convenient, affordable, and mainstream. These ripple effects and positive feedback loops make meat reduction at the individual level even more meaningful in the long term.

WHEN A GLOBAL CATASTROPHE STRIKES

David Denkenberger

Author of *Feeding Everyone No Matter What: Managing Food Security after Global Catastrophe*

We live in a world that is at risk. An asteroid or comet impact or a large volcanic eruption could obscure the sun. Nuclear war could cause the burning of cities and an atmosphere full of smoke. Increased climate change activity could cause a 10°C (18°F) regional temperature shift, with devastating consequences. A super pest, pathogen, or weed could emerge that destroys crops. There could also be a breakdown of the international food trade caused by a pandemic or conventional world war. In all of these scenarios—one or more of which is likely to happen in the next hundred years—global stores of food will be essential. Eating less meat could mean fewer animals and less grain stored. And yet, it would be a mistake to use this as an argument against curtailing overall meat consumption. Ultimately, the advantages of eating less meat will outweigh any potential detrimental outcomes that might be occurring during periods of catastrophe.

Let's first take a step back and examine this problem in the context of the very long view. Many people, myself included, are not just concerned about the people who will live in this century. Philosophically, the day or year you are born should not determine how much your life is worth. From this perspective, planning for the far future is overwhelmingly important. Even if you don't believe that we will colonize the galaxy or upload our brains into computers, we could very well be living on Earth for many, many more generations. We need to start thinking now about how we are going to sustain those lives.

All of this is to say, I understand people who argue we shouldn't try to reduce our meat consumption because it may hurt our ability to respond to global catastrophes. However, there is a way out. It turns out that there is a far more effective way to prepare for global agricultural catastrophes than simply storing more food. This strategy hinges on something known as alternate food, or foods that depend on stored biomass or fossil fuels as energy sources, like specialized forms of natural-gas loving bacteria. While eating bacteria may not sound appealing, we actually already do. The common dietary supplement spirulina is actually cyanobacteria, and it is generally recognized that mitochondria and chloroplasts are captured bacteria that power animal and plant cells, respectively.

Another strategy involves planning for possible events, notably a decrease in sunlight. If the sun is blocked for some reason, humans need to be ready to adapt. One big change in such a scenario would be an increase in dead trees. While not aesthetically pleasing, dead trees can be consumed directly by organisms like mushrooms and some beetles. Other animals, including cattle, sheep, goats, horses, deer, and rats, could eat the wood after it had been softened by mushrooms. In natural ecosystems, fish will eat leaves, not because they can digest fiber, but because they can digest the bacteria rotting the leaves. This technique could also work as chicken feed. The vast majority of current biofuels consume human edible food. However, there are cellulosic or second-generation biofuels that turn fiber into sugar and then sugar into ethanol. In a real food catastrophe, we could just eat the sugar.

Storing enough food for years of consumption would be extremely expensive, costing trillions of dollars. However, it would only cost tens of millions of dollars to significantly increase our chances of feeding everyone in a global catastrophe through alternate food experimentation. Therefore, you can offset the slight increase in global catastrophic risk due to consuming less meat by supporting alternate food efforts. Overall, the advantages of eating less meat will offset the downsides.

AN UNCERTAIN PHOSPHORUS FUTURE

▊ Will Brownlie

Researcher at the Centre of Ecology and Hydrology, University of Edinburgh

Currently we cannot feed the population without using fertilizers. This is indisputably a bad thing. Driven by our unsustainable use of fertilizers in food production and our increasing consumption of foods with big phosphorus footprints—predominantly meat—we may be approaching a global tipping point. If no action is taken to curb our unsustainable use of phosphorus, our future ability to produce sufficient food to feed the population, maintain clean and safe water resources and ecosystems, and manage international conflicts arising from uneven phosphorus distribution is in jeopardy.

Phosphorus (P)—along with nitrogen (N) and potassium (K)—is one of the three essential components of fertilizer and cannot be substituted by any other element. As the global demand for food increases, so will the demand for fertilizer—especially phosphorus. Indeed, dealing with the consequences of our currently unsustainable use of phosphorus may become one of the most crucial social and environmental challenges of this century.

THE IMPACTS OF UNSUSTAINABLE PHOSPHORUS USE

The mining of phosphorus at first seemed to be a smart decision. By facilitating bigger and bigger harvests, it has supported exponential population growth (estimated to reach 9.2 billion by 2050). For some countries, the sudden boost in availability of phosphorus did indeed provide prosperity. However, countries without easy access to phosphorus have grown reliant on imports. This means mining the finite phosphorus rock reserves has created a bubble. We now have a population that simply cannot be fed without access to more phosphorus, even as the average amount of phosphorus needed per individual is increasing. This last part is, in large part, because of meat.

Over the last fifty years, the average amount of meat and the caloric intake of the human diet have substantially increased. This dietary change has subsequently raised the average global human phosphorus footprint by 38 percent, with meat consumption accounting for 72 percent of the global average individual's phosphorus footprint.[1]

Simply put, meat production is no longer an efficient way of meeting human dietary needs. Currently, producing a unit of meat protein takes up to ten times the resources (not just in phosphorus) of producing vegetarian proteins. And the entire process is incredibly wasteful, from mining wastage, inefficient agricultural practices, and even wasted food. For example, we are currently using vast amounts of phosphorus to grow food to feed our livestock. And yet, we could be using this phosphorus to grow crops to feed ourselves directly. In comparison, the phosphorus used to make one eight-ounce steak is the same amount used to grow 755 potatoes.

The problem doesn't end with the types of food we eat, however. The planet currently manages to produce enough food to feed everybody, but the bounty is not being equally shared. The world hosts 868 million undernourished people, with 36 million people dying each year from starvation. But it also supports the diets of 1.5 billion obese or overweight individuals. Of these, 29 people will die each year because they eat too much food.

DO WE HAVE ENOUGH PHOSPHORUS LEFT FOR EVERYONE?

Our current global reliance on phosphorus would be less intimidating if each country had a limitless supply of the resource's rock deposits or even if we recycled the same amount of phosphorus that we used up. Unfortunately, only a handful of countries supply phosphorus for the rest of the globe. It is estimated that around 74 percent of identified phosphorus rock reserves are located in Morocco or occupied Western Sahara. Meanwhile, current U.S. mineral reserves will run out in the next thirty years. Western Europe and India are almost completely dependent on phosphorus imports.

The European Union has already placed phosphate rock on its critical raw materials list. Potential political instability in phosphorus-exporting countries is also threatening global accessibility.

While some people have compared our global shortage of phosphorus to the limited global reserves of oil, it's an imperfect metaphor. If we run out of oil, we can make energy from wind and sunlight. But the use of phosphorus in fertilizer cannot be substituted by any other element. We are talking about nothing short of a long-term global threat.

Of most immediate concern are the fluctuating fertilizer prices driven by decreasing phosphorus rock quality and political instability. Diminishing rock quality has been observed in practically all such reserves. When quality goes down, it makes extraction more expensive, increasing the price of fertilizer and consequently of food. We saw the full scope of this threat in 2008, when a peak in phosphorus fertilizer price was linked to a global increase in food prices, resulting in riots across the world. It is not surprising that the most economically disadvantaged populations are at the biggest risk. Food security is now linked to phosphorus security, and this means ensuring all farmers have sufficient access.

PHOSPHORUS AND THE ENVIRONMENT

The problems don't stop with food insecurity, however. Our unsustainable use of phosphorus is also harming our environment. The release of phosphorus previously stored underground has profoundly disrupted freshwater ecosystems, many of which are now full of much more phosphorus than they can cope with. Once in the water supply, phosphorus runoff can cause rapid and harmful algal blooms. Basically, the algal populations have all the components they need to grow (that is, water, carbon, light, and nitrogen). When threshold phosphorus concentration is reached, rapid algal blooms can turn healthy freshwaters into toxic green bogs. This can occur almost overnight, leaving waters so deoxygenated that fish and plants suffocate. The process, termed *eutrophication*, is the single greatest cause of water quality deterioration globally. The combined costs of water treatment and restoration, coupled with losses incurred by local economies, have been estimated at $2.2 billion per year.[2]

THE ROLE OF THE INDIVIDUAL IN THE GLOBAL P CYCLE

Up to now, efforts to reduce phosphorus accumulation in the environment have focused on increasing agricultural efficiency and recycling phosphorus from wastes. But these strategies alone will not achieve sustainability. Improving the behavior of the consumer is as important as improving the behavior of the producers. The human phosphorus cycle is mainly driven by meat consumption, making individual lifestyle choices an important part of any solution. And yet, it is important that any aspirational goals must be achievable.

Effective long-term strategies to help fix unsustainable resource use will require cultural and behavioral shifts in attitude. Governments can build environmental policies that will help phosphorus-use efficiency, but in a growing climate of short-term political agenda, we need to remember that change can also be achieved through small individual acts. A challenging future lies ahead, one in which global resources will be needed to support the largest human population the planet has ever seen. The odds may be long, but they are not impossible. Already, people across the planet are doing their part by following a simple maxim: "It is not necessarily about not eating meat; it is about eating less meat."

TIPPING THE ENERGY SCALES

■ Dale Jamieson

Author of *Reason in a Dark Time: Why the Struggle against Climate Change Failed—and What It Means for Our Future*

Everything we do requires energy, but not all energy is created the same way. Some energy comes from the burning of fossil fuels, while eating fruits and nuts creates an entirely different power source. What every way of producing energy has in common, however, is the inherent transformation of nature. Just like with the energy sources themselves, not all of these transformations are created equally: Burning fossil fuels disrupts the climate, something researchers believe will eventually kill millions of people and cause untold damages. Luckily, there are ways to minimize this destructive fossil fuel consumption. One of the simplest is to cut down on our daily meat intake.

Here's a practical, real-world example. Suppose you want to go to the store to buy food. Driving to the store requires energy, but so does walking. It is surprising that if you have an extremely fuel-efficient car and a terrible meat-heavy diet, you could actually use less energy driving to the store than walking to it. Walking may be good exercise, but depending on your diet, it is better for the climate if we drive in certain situations.

This seemingly paradoxical result is a consequence of meat-loving America's long, energy-intensive, massively inefficient supply chain. Consider the egalitarian cheeseburger: Each burger requires a tremendous amount of grain to be fed to cows; cows happen to be terrible at turning grain into beef. In fact, it takes approximately sixteen pounds of grain and 2,000 gallons of water to produce one measly pound of meat.

Growing the grain to feed the cows is itself a massively energy-intensive, inefficient process. Farm machinery runs mostly on fossil fuels: grain, meat, fertilizer, and pesticides all must be transported, and the agricultural workers must be fed. Meanwhile, cows and fertilizer manufacturing contribute methane to the atmosphere as well as carbon dioxide. As it happens, methane is a greater immediate threat to the climate than carbon dioxide. As a greenhouse gas, methane is 25 percent times more potent than carbon dioxide. (Fortunately, it has a shorter lifespan in the atmosphere.) Returning to our walking vs. driving conundrum, our bodies are even less efficient in converting calories than an internal combustion engine. All of which is to say, it takes a lot of carbon to make a car, but burning gasoline is not as hostile to the climate as eating beef.

This is not an absolute rule, of course. The numbers vary greatly depending on a variety of factors, including if your car is a gas-guzzler. In situations like this, getting your beef-fueled body to the store on foot may be the more efficient option. Obviously, the calculations also turn out differently if you are vegan. Vegans should pretty much always walk to the store, even if they own a Prius.

For those of us who care about the environment, these types of calculations serve as a reminder that our eating habits have consequences. Don't want to wrestle with the awkwardness of having to figure out whether it's better to drive or walk? Why not try veganism for at least part of the time and set your mind at ease? Ultimately, no matter what we eat, biking is always more efficient than either driving or walking. The moral of this story is reduce your meat consumption, get a bike—and never forget to enjoy life.

REPLENISHING A THIRSTY PLANET

■ Wendy Pabich

Author of *Taking on Water: How One Water Expert Challenged Her Inner Hypocrite, Reduced Her Water Footprint (without Sacrificing a Toasty Shower), and Found Nirvana*

Water is getting scarce. Recent years have brought extreme drought, low snow packs, and some of the lowest stream flows on record for a number of river systems. We see Las Vegas waging water war with the open ranch lands to the north; Atlanta, Georgia, is in protracted battles with downstream states over its primary water supply at Lake Lanier; and water tables beneath California's San Joaquin Valley—the source of 40 percent of the nation's fruits and vegetables—are dropping. A recent study by the Natural Resources Defense Council suggests that by mid-century, half the counties in the United States will be facing water scarcity. These problems are not going away anytime soon.

To begin with, the global population has grown to over 7 billion people and demand for water has escalated. Today, we use water not only for basic needs like food preparation, drinking water, and sanitation but also to produce power and manufacture untold consumer goods. The growing global demand for food and consumer goods is putting tremendous pressure on water resources, lessening the volume, quality, and consistency of available water, and causing a loss of biodiversity and resiliency in ecosystems of all types. Water overuse, river fragmentation, the draining of wetlands, and pollution are all diminishing the ability of these systems to provide a range of ecosystem services—flood control, clean drinking water, clean air, habitat, decomposition of wastes, food production, pharmaceuticals, and recreational and spiritual benefits.

We often think of our individual water use as encompassing a few necessary, daily categories like drinking, cooking, bathing, cleaning, and tending our lawns. On average, Americans each use about 100 gallons of water per day—or 36,500 gallons per year— for these purposes. Yet, this water use is only the tip of the iceberg. We also use water indirectly because water is "embedded" in the products and services we buy. Thus, in the same way we each have a carbon footprint, we also have a water footprint.

A water footprint is the total volume of freshwater used directly and indirectly to produce the goods and services consumed by an individual, community, company, or nation. This includes the amount of "green water" (rainwater) consumed in the production process and used to grow crops as well as the "blue water" (surface and groundwater) consumed, and "gray water," the amount of freshwater polluted as a result of the process.

To put this in perspective, a cup of coffee requires about 37 gallons of water to produce, as compared to the nearly 2,000 gallons of water used to produce one pound of beef or the 2,200 gallons used to create a pair of blue jeans. About 25 gallons can produce a kilowatt-hour of electricity. Estimates vary, but data from the Water Footprint Network suggests that the annual water footprint of the average American consumer is more than 750,000 gallons per year, nearly 60 percent of which is used in the production of our food. By contrast, nations like Guatemala, Kenya, and Afghanistan have water footprints measuring less than 200,000 gallons per person per year.

The meat on our dinner plates takes a tremendous amount of water to produce. In the United States, agriculture accounts for some 80 percent of our country's consumptive water use. According to the Water Footprint Network, about 1,799 gallons of water are used to produce one pound of beef, 468 gallons per pound of chicken, 576 gallons per pound of pork, and 880 gallons per gallon of milk. Copious volumes of water are also needed to grow feed for animals, while additional, albeit smaller, amounts are used to care for animals, process meat, and distribute and sell animal products.

In contrast, raising vegetables and grains requires a fraction of the water: Carrots require 6.5 gallons of water per pound; an apple uses 18 gallons of water; peas use 10.2 gallons per pound; blueberries use 13.8 gallons per cup; and potatoes use 119 gallons per pound.

Our meat-heavy diet is therefore bad for our health but also bad for our water supplies and our land. Studies suggest that shifting toward a vegetarian diet could reduce our national food-related water footprint by more than a third. This does not mean we all need to become vegetarian, however; incremental changes matter. By avoiding meat for two days a week, you can reduce your water footprint by about 950 gallons. Spread out over a year, this practice can save nearly 50,000 gallons. If we implemented this strategy as a nation, we could save nearly 160 trillion gallons of water.

Similarly, wasting food wastes water. A recent study in the UK calculated that embedded water in food waste within the country accounted for one and a half times the volume of water people actually used in their homes. Estimates of U.S. food waste range from 14 to 50 percent of all food produced for domestic sale and consumption. It is important that more than one quarter of all meat produced for the retail market goes to waste. Much of this food is tossed in the garbage because it has passed its sell-by date (often mistakenly identified as the date food should be eaten by), is no longer considered fresh, or was simply allowed to spoil, often due to overpurchasing. It is estimated that fully one quarter of U.S. water consumption is used to produce this wasted food. By not wasting food this week—particularly water-intensive meat and dairy—you can reduce your water footprint by about 667 gallons. By continuing this practice, you can save nearly 35,000 gallons of water in a year. And, again, the collective impact is significant. As a nation, we could save nearly 112 trillion gallons of water, just by being a little more mindful.

THE HUMANE MEAT MYTH

James McWilliams

Author of *The Modern Savage: Our Unthinking Decision to Eat Animals*

Reducing our agricultural footprint on the planet is frequently portrayed as an immensely complicated task to achieve. In fact, at least as a theoretical matter, it's remarkably simple: We need to radically curtail our consumption of animal products.

Of course, theory is one thing, reality quite another. In reality, the challenge is far more burdensome. Eschewing animal products in a culture that largely celebrates eating animals can be, at best, socially awkward and, at worst, ostracizing. The pervasive pro–meat social context that marks our reality is an intransigent baseline for change, and the challenge it poses should not be downplayed. Humans are inherently social creatures—we want to be invited to dinner! But if consumer behavior is going to have a meaningful impact on global ecology, much less on animal welfare, the vast majority of us will have to participate in the project of reducing (and eventually ending) our reliance on the meat and dairy industries. The vast majority of us, in other words, will somehow have to opt out of the traditional system.

A small but vocal group of food reformers suggests that, despite these challenges, important changes are already afoot. The so-called food movement seeks to avoid industrially produced animal goods, preferring to eat from small farms practicing more humane and sustainable methods of production. Whereas vegans—who, it should be noted, exist on the periphery of the food movement—urge the complete avoidance of animal products, members of the food movement believe we can in fact continue to eat animals, just as long as they are from the right kind of farms.

This position is extremely popular, and for good reason. For one, it makes intuitive sense—animals are usually treated better on nonindustrial farms than they are on factory farms. And on the surface it would appear that nonindustrial farms are less polluting than their industrial counterparts. For another, it requires a smaller sacrifice—thereby pragmatically improving the odds that people will sign on.

For all the attention the alternative position generates, however, it may be a counterproductive approach to reducing the harm done to domesticated animals. I realize that this claim sounds counterintuitive. If buying from nonindustrial farms rather than industrial ones represents a decline in suffering, how is there not a net gain? Unfortunately, it may not be that simple.

Let's begin with what I think is an irrefutable premise: Consumers en masse will always tend to buy the cheapest animal products on the market. Even if a small percentage—or even a large minority—choose the more humane and thus more expensive option, the bulk of consumers will continue to support the less expensive, more industrial option. (Note: according to every measure, producing meat and dairy with sustainable and humane methods raises the cost of production.) Given this reality, the option of supporting the nonindustrial alternative fails to question the legitimacy of eating animals. As the global population grows, and as the basic act of eating animals is reiterated as culturally acceptable, supporting humane and sustainable alternatives may end up being worse than irrelevant—it could (inadvertently) encourage consumption from factory farms.

But what if you could wave a magic wand and make all animal farms into nonindustrial operations that employed the highest ethical and ecological standards? Would that solve the problem of widespread suffering among domesticated farm animals? Again, against all intuitions, the answer is probably no. Provided that consumers en masse prefer the cheapest option and provided that it is always cheaper to produce animal products through industrial methods, capitalism would take over. With competition for market share would come a creeping incentive to cut corners. Ambitious farms would reduce welfare measures, expand, seek economies of scale, and inevitably reach the level of an industrial operation. In over ten years of making this argument, I have yet to hear a viable reason proving it could be theoretically wrong.

Unfortunately, this probably leaves the consumer who wants to affect agrarian change with virtuous food choices stranded. On the one hand, it's obvious to declare that we should forget reducing meat consumption and "go vegan." There is no doubt that a global transition to veganism would have radically positive implications for animals and the health of the planet. But slogans are easy. The very prospect of such a transition, in light of our current support for eating animals, borders on the absurd. This leaves the matter in the hands of you and me.

Fortunately, despite the severity and extent of the problem, we can foster genuine change in a seemingly intractable food system without condemning ourselves to social Siberia. Consumer power—voting with your fork—is easy to overstate. But we can and must make ethical shifts in consumer behavior by limiting our intake of animal products (no matter what the source). In and of themselves, these changes won't make a revolution. But, inevitably, they have the potential to initiate a new evolution by becoming visible for others to witness and providing the raw material for a culinary foundation that, one day, will see eating animals as the remnant of a less enlightened past.

FOOD FROM THE SEA

█ Nancy Knowlton

Author of *Citizens of the Sea: Wondrous Creatures from the
Census of Marine Life*

For years the ocean was thought to be limitless in its ability to feed
humanity. After all, it covers over 70 percent of the surface of the
planet and its deep waters represent over 95 percent of the earth's
habitable real estate. Nevertheless, over time, fishing effort has in-
tensified dramatically, and new technologies have made it vastly
easier to find and catch fish. The result has been the removal of
most of the large fish from the sea.

As a young scientist, I experienced this firsthand on the coral
reefs of Jamaica. When I first arrived, the corals were thriving, but
the extreme scarcity of fish was immediately apparent. Poor fishers
without the guidance of a plan for fishing sustainably had stripped
these reefs of anything big. At the time we didn't realize the danger
this posed, but we soon learned the hard way that coral reefs need
their fish to stay healthy. Without seaweed-eating fish, the seaweeds eventually overgrew and smothered the corals. It's not just
corals that depend on healthy fish communities. In the north Atlantic, kelp forests without cod and other large bottom-dwelling
fish experience explosions of sea urchins that in turn decimate the
kelp, creating wastelands of nearly bare rock.

In some cases our harvesting methods compound the problem
of overfishing itself. On coral reefs fringing the coasts of developing countries, fishers using dynamite or cyanide have killed vast
areas of once living coral. The industrial analog is trawling, which
is essentially the strip mining of the sea floor. Bycatch, the inad-
vertent killing of noncommercial species, has taken a large toll on
seabirds and other marine life that are attracted to baited hooks or
ensnared in nets.

In fact, our appetite for seafood has been so intense for so long
that we have forgotten what marine ecosystems looked like before

they were so heavily harvested. Green sea turtles used to be so numerous that they kept sea grasses cropped short like golf courses, but when the turtles were hunted to near extinction, the sea grass beds became stagnant and prone to disease. In estuaries like the Chesapeake Bay, oysters in huge numbers used to filter the water, keeping it clean and clear. Today one has to travel to extremely remote or very well protected locations to get a glimpse of what ocean ecosystems used to look like before we arrived on the scene. On reefs surrounding uninhabited atolls of the central Pacific, the waters teem with turtles, manta rays, snappers, groupers, and sharks.

Clearly our demand for seafood has outstripped the capacity of the sea to provide it. How then can we get our relationship with Planet Ocean back in balance? Choices about what and how much we take from the sea are vital in this regard. Sylvia Earle, renowned spokesperson for the ocean, simply eats no seafood at all. But even land food often draws from the sea thanks to the multitude of uses for fishmeal, for example. Moreover, there are important health benefits associated with a diet whose protein is derived from seafood. What follows is what I think about when making seafood choices.

Some forms of sea life reproduce quickly, while others reproduce slowly. One of the reasons sharks have been so harmed by demand for their fins is that many bear only a small number of live young at a time. Many deep-sea fish, like orange roughy, have lifespans that rival our own. The slower the reproductive rate, the longer it takes for populations to recover from harvesting.

Routinely eating low on the ocean food chain is a good idea because every step up the food chain represents a substantial loss of energy. On land, it is no accident that the vast majority of animals we raise to eat consume plants. In the sea, aquaculture of organisms that eat plants or filter tiny animals and plants from plankton has less of an impact on ocean ecosystems than does aquaculture of predatory fish, like salmon, that are fed fish. The same principle holds for wild-caught seafood, but we do need to remember that other organisms depend on "forage fish" like sardines and herring for dinner. Seaweeds are at the very bottom of the food chain (and are delicious), though as with any aquaculture or harvesting, damage can be done when it is not well managed.

Some fish play extremely important roles that influence entire ecosystems. Seaweed-eating fish, like parrotfish, are essential for healthy coral reefs, which is why bans on fishing for parrotfish are increasing, despite the fact that as plant eaters they are close to the bottom of the food chain. Conversely, eating of invasive species, like predatory lionfish in the Caribbean, can be done ecologically guilt free because they have very negative impacts on these reefs.

There is also human welfare to consider. Where tourism is an important contributor to the local economy, sea life is often more valuable alive than on the plate. Bans on shark finning have been established around the world, not only because their numbers have been so depleted but also because tourists pay a lot of money to see them swimming underwater. In Palau it has been estimated that a dead shark is worth $108 but a live shark is worth $1.9 million over the course of its lifetime.

Finally, there are ethical choices associated with eating any animal life, and the marine animals that humans eat span a wide range of mental capacities. Marine mammals like whales and dolphins are highly intelligent, with complex social systems. Octopuses also have large brains and sophisticated behaviors, which is why they are covered by animal care regulations in Europe. At the other end of the spectrum, organisms like oysters, mussels, sea cucumbers, and sea urchins have little in the way of what we would call a brain.

In sum, it's complicated, and an ocean-savvy consumer needs to stay informed. Eating of fish that are sustainably harvested through gear or harvest regulations or the establishment of marine protected areas is far preferable to eating fish, like blue-fin tuna, whose numbers remain far below historical levels. Some types of aquaculture have minimal impact on the ocean, others not so much. Perhaps the most important rules of thumb when it comes to eating seafood are the same as they are for food from the land: Waste not, and moderation in all things.

THE NITROGEN STORY

▌ Mark A. Sutton

NERC Centre for Ecology & Hydrology and honorary professor at the University of Edinburgh

▌ Clare M. Howard

NERC Centre for Ecology & Hydrology and the University of Edinburgh

If you like to breathe clean air, drink safe water, reduce your impact on biodiversity, and keep soils healthy, then reducing your meat consumption not only makes sense but nets you multiple brownie points in the process.

To begin, we need to first understand where nitrogen comes from and why we use so much of it. Nitrogen is an essential nutrient for plant growth—like it or loathe it, we need to work with the nitrogen cycle to grow vegetables and cereals as well as to feed livestock. Around 78 percent of our atmosphere is made up of nitrogen in the form of dinitrogen gas (N_2); we breathe this kind of nitrogen constantly. However, this is an unreactive form of nitrogen—it does not harm humans, but it is also in the wrong form to effectively aid growth. Plants need nitrogen in a reactive form such as ammonia (NH_3), ammonium (NH_4), or nitrate (NO_3). Such forms can be found in animal manures. They are also manufactured by humans to be used as synthetic fertilizers, similar to what you can buy in a garden supply store. Unfortunately, reactive nitrogen has a negative impact on the environment.

The history of nitrogen is a checkered one—besides its more benign use as a source of plant nutrients, nitrogen is also a key component in some explosives. For many years, the chemical element was quite hard to find—humans tried everything, from mining bird poop islands in Peru to collecting saltpeter from the Atacama Desert in northern Chile. This all changed with Fritz Haber's discovery in 1908 of a new manufacturing technique. Suddenly, engineers were able to extract ammonia from the air. Soon, Carl Bosch invented a complementary process that allowed Haber's technique to be implemented on an industrial scale. Almost overnight the human race had greatly increased its abilities to prevent hunger—and destroy its enemies.

Today, it is estimated that around half of all humans owe their existence to synthetic fertilizers. Estimating the number of people who have perished at the hands of explosives in the past 100 or so years is more difficult, but the numbers must surely number in the tens of millions.

But human aggression is not the only problem exacerbated by nitrogen. As with many activities, the use of nitrogen in farming is inefficient. Inevitably, reactive nitrogen is released into the air as ammonia and greenhouse gas nitrous oxide (N_2O); it may also seep into the water in the form of nitrate. In some cases, as much as 80 percent of the nitrogen used is being lost to pollution.[1]

Eating meat causes higher emissions of nitrogen pollutants than eating vegetables and cereals. This is partly because of the long production chain needed to raise livestock—between the grain needed to fatten the animals and the manure produced, it would actually be more efficient to eat the animal feed. In fact, scientific estimates from Europe suggest that fully 85 percent of the nitrogen yield of harvested crops goes to feed livestock.

Once the reactive nitrogen has been released into the air and water, it moves through the system in a number of ways. As nitrate, it affects the quality of drinking water, potentially impacting rates of heart disease and cancer. It also stimulates excessive algae growth in bodies of water, sucking up all the oxygen and leading to death of the fish. Nitrogen from fertilizers and manures is released into the air as ammonia. On a local scale, ammonia has a toxic effect on sensitive plant species—not to mention the smell. Further afield, ammonia contributes to the formation of very fine particles suspended in the air known as particulate matter. These can travel thousands of miles from the source, increasing the risk of heart and lung problems as well as cancer.

If that all wasn't bad enough, the process of farming itself releases nitrous oxide into the air. Perhaps better known as laughing gas, nitrous oxide (N_2O) is a greenhouse gas 300 times stronger than carbon dioxide. N_2O contributes to the thinning of our planet's vital protective ozone. This layer prevents the sun's harmful ultraviolet radiation from reaching Earth's surface. The banning of chlorofluorocarbons (CFCs) was an important step in the right direction but nitrous oxide remains a major problem in terms of ozone depletion. It is no laughing matter.

So what kind of a difference could reducing your meat intake really have? In Europe, scientists have been asking themselves this very same question. Their findings show that if Europeans were to reduce their meat intake by 50 percent, polluting emissions would drop by around 40 percent.[2] This is not a bad return on your emotional investment.

However, it is important to pay attention to the details of any dietary changes. Switching from chargrilled meat to cheese at dinner will help, of course, but it would be even better to replace your meat entrée with vegetables or cereals. In other words: less of the steak and more of the sweet corn.

Ultimately, the agriculture business is partially responsible for the problem—and also has the power to be part of the solution. Improved techniques in the use and storage of manures and fertilizers will help decrease air and water pollution, for example. A group of creative scientists have also been experimenting with more out-of-the-box solutions. For example, scientists have developed a robotic "terminator" designed to kill an insidious coral-eating starfish known as crown-of-thorns. The species, which has been taking over coral reefs, multiplies quickly in water polluted by nitrogen-rich farm runoff.

The terminator invention is a testament to the determination of scientists, but not all solutions need to be this complicated. This is where the reducetarian method comes into play: Eat less meat (and eggs and dairy), and increase the amount of fruit and vegetables that you eat. After all, if you were filling a leaky bucket and your shoes were getting wet, the first thing to do would be to turn off the tap—not try to redesign the bucket (or your shoes).

THE FALSE DICHOTOMY OF LIVING WELL AND LIVING GENTLY

Naomi Oreskes

Co-author of *The Collapse of Western Civilization: A View from the Future*

Back in the 1980s, I used to work in the mining industry. At the time, some of my colleagues drove cars emblazoned with bumper stickers that read: "Let the bastards freeze in the dark!" The "bastards," of course, were the environmentalists and liberal politicians trying to stop the mining industry from running roughshod over the environment. The laws passed during this time were a crucial part of the effort to clean up America's skies and waterways, preserving biodiversity and protecting our nation's unique natural beauty. They tried to force the industry to correct its foolish ways, and in some respects, it worked. America continued to be a prosperous country, but also a far safer and more beautiful one. And none of us have frozen in the dark.

Still, the sentiments expressed by those 1980s bumper stickers haven't exactly gone away. We still face a seemingly dichotomous choice, between living well and living gently. We are told that if we want to be comfortable, our natural environment must pay the price. To cite just one example: Recently, I was accused on Twitter of being a hypocrite for supporting fossil fuel divestment. The critic argued that without those fuels, I and my fellow Massachusetts residents would have all frozen this past winter.

This, of course, is ridiculous: People found a way to live through plenty of harsh winters before the widespread use of fossil fuels. Americans in the seventeenth, eighteenth, and nineteenth centuries had heat and they had light. (Native Americans did too.) What fossil fuels did for New Englanders—and for people around the globe— was to make heat and light more accessible, more convenient, and cheaper. They also made life more fun. In the early twentieth century, coal-powered electricity lit up the midtown Manhattan's Great White Way and powered trolleys that took people to amusement parks. A few decades later, cheap gasoline was enabling people to take "Sunday drives" to green spaces outside of the hot and crowded cities. When I was a child, my family's summer vacations were car trips: We saw the United States through the glass windows of our Chevrolet—or sometimes a rented Ford station wagon. And it was a good ride, while it lasted.

But what we have learned in recent decades is this kind of access and fun come with a hidden price. The external costs of fossil fuels are diverse, but the single greatest threat facing the world as a whole is climate change. Scientists around the globe have proven time and time again that the world is warming rapidly, and greenhouse gases produced by fossil fuels are to blame. Alarming changes in the world's physical, chemical and biological environment are under way. To stop these changes completely will require profound shifts in the way we live, and this worries many people, no matter what their political persuasion. Folks inside the fossil fuel industry remain comfortable ignoring reality, but even for those not in denial, some people seem concerned that environmentally friendly policies could make our way of life less comfortable.

Personally, I think this last concern is at best misplaced, and at worst a myth being quietly pushed by the fossil fuel industry. In the long run, to be sure, we need to eliminate fossil fuels almost entirely. This will mean a large-scale transformation of our energy system. But in the short run, we can do a lot simply by reducing our use. The average Californian uses about 30 percent less energy than other Americans, and life there is pretty darn good. Some of that difference is due to the state's mild climate, but not all of it. California has spent years enacting sensible policies that encourage energy efficiency, while promoting a culture of mindfulness about environmental protection. And you don't have to live in a warm place to benefit from energy efficiency: Germans use about the same amount of energy as Californians, and they are quite warm and snug in their homes in winter.

It turns out a great deal of energy use is just habit. Some changes, like changing our light bulbs or making sure that our car tires are properly inflated, are easy. If we want to go further, however, it might not hurt to get creative. A few years ago, when I was living in southern California, we had an electricity outage on a Friday afternoon. My neighborhood organized an impromptu picnic on the street—people shared food and drink, and, as the stars came out, we stayed up late, chatting, bonding, and generally having a good time. By the end of the evening, the entire block was discussing the idea of an "electricity-free Friday." By morning, the lights were back on and by Monday the idea had been forgotten.

But why not do it? Many people now practice Meatless Mondays, which are a win–win–win–win. It's better for the environment, it's better for our health, lots of vegetarian food tastes delicious, and it almost always costs less to eat vegetables than to eat meat. Reducing doesn't automatically mean suffering, it just means reorganizing, often in ways that ultimately pay dividends. Just as some people have reduced their meat consumption by eliminating meat at breakfast or lunch, an electricity-free Friday doesn't have to last the whole day, it could just be an evening. Next Friday night, try turning off the TV, the radio, the computer, and the phones, lighting some candles, making a vegetable crudité platter or other food that doesn't require cooking, and just spending the night talking. Come winter, you could light a fire or snuggle up in bed. That doesn't sound like suffering to me.

THROUGH ALIEN EYES

■ Nigel Henbest

Co-author of *The Astronomy Bible: The Definitive Guide to the Night Sky and the Universe*

■ Heather Couper

Co-author of *The Astronomy Bible: The Definitive Guide to the Night Sky and the Universe*

There's huge excitement in the astronomy world. Researchers have discovered intelligent life on a planet—not just one kind of alien being, but several. But they are baffled by what kind of morality—if any—reigns on this world.

The first aliens they found were the Gips, a peaceful race that lives in the woods and eats fruit and nuts. But then scientists were confronted with the cruel race of the Namuhs. They habitually kill each other, often in the most brutal ways.

These bloodthirsty aliens seem to have a vendetta against the peaceful Gips, not only killing them painfully but then dismembering the bodies and actually eating the dead Gips.

Investigating further, scientists have identified horrendous concentration camps, where the Namuhs have imprisoned the gentle Gips and then execute them—thousands at a time. Horrifically, the Namuhs then celebrate by feasting off the corpses.

Where is this "alien world"? Not in some far-flung region of the cosmos, in fact. What we've described is our own planet Earth: just reverse the word *Gip* to make "Pig" and *Namuh* to become "Human," and you can see how the inhabitants of our world would seem to an intelligent and dispassionate visitor, with our cruel farming methods and appalling abattoirs.

As lifelong astronomers, we've grown accustomed to taking literally the broadest perspective, when it comes to understanding what's going on here on Earth. And the grandstand view from space does make you see many of the traditions of terrestrial cultures in a new light.

Apollo astronaut Ed Mitchell described the Earth as "a sparkling blue and white jewel; a light, delicate sky-blue sphere laced with slowly swirling veils of white . . . like a small pearl in a thick sea of black mystery."

It's difficult to reconcile that idyllic vision with the scenes of misery, depravity, and carnage that are actually to be found in our planet.

We have both been long-term vegetarians—Heather since the age of four—as well as astronomers from childhood. After the early excitement of being a kid, out alone late at night with a telescope, gazing all alone at planets, stars, and nebulae, we each elected to take our first degrees in astrophysics, at the University of Leicester—where we met.

Heather went on to conduct research at Oxford, while Nigel moved to the radio astronomy department at Cambridge. Here, there had recently been a "scare" about aliens. Jocelyn Bell and Tony Hewish had found regular pulses of radio waves coming from an object deep in space. The signal looked suspiciously artificial. The researchers—half jokingly—labeled it LGM, for little green men.

The department head, Martin Ryle, was seriously worried. If the pulses proved to be from alien life, he said, "Burn the records and forget about this, because if the news gets out that there is intelligence out there people will want to launch a signal in that direction to talk to them." If the aliens were "looking for a planet to occupy the next thing that will happen is that we will be invaded."

These "signals" turned out to be natural. They are radio waves from a tiny star—a neutron star, or pulsar—that is spinning rapidly, and the radiation sweeps past the Earth in regular bursts, like the beam from a lighthouse.

But Ryle's prediction of humans drawing attention to planet Earth was spot-on. In 1974, American astronomer Frank Drake used the world's largest radio telescope—at Arecibo in Puerto Rico—to transmit a message to the cosmos. It described human biology and anatomy and included a map showing how to locate planet Earth.

Ryle wrote an impassioned letter to Drake, deploring his action. Ryle declared it was "very hazardous to reveal our existence and location to the Galaxy; for all we know, any creatures out there might be malevolent—or hungry."

Hungry aliens—fortunately fictional!—did feature in the 1962 television production "To Serve Man," part of *The Twilight Zone* science fiction series. A book on board a visiting UFO is titled *To Serve Man*, but—as the hero gruesomely discovers at the end—it's not a guide to helping mankind but is instead a cookbook.

But would aliens really want to eat us?

The people who have pondered longest and deepest on the nature and motivation of intelligent aliens are the scientists involved in the Search for Extraterrestrial Intelligence (SETI). They cover a huge range of expertise, from anthropology and biology to philosophy and—of course—the technology that's required to seek out a radio message or laser signal that's traveled over thousands of light-years of space on its way to us from ET.

The father of SETI, Frank Drake—who's been searching for alien broadcasts for over fifty years—believes that any civilization advanced enough to send interstellar signals and to travel the galaxy must have overcome the belligerence that afflicts a stripling race like humans.

His colleague Dan Werthimer elaborates. "I think it's likely that advanced civilizations are going to be peaceful," he's told us, "because the ones that are not so peaceful are going to blow themselves up, and they're not going to be around anymore. I don't think they're killing each other the way we are."

He pointedly adds: "I don't think other civilizations are going to come and eat us."

It makes total sense. Though we might not know exactly what the little green men would put on their preferred menus, we do know a lot about what one particular intelligent species thinks: people here on planet Earth.

Over decades of public presentations, we have been asked literally a thousand times whether there is life elsewhere in the universe. It's way ahead of the other popular questions: What happened before the Big Bang; and what would happen if I fell into a black hole?

And it's a positive interest. People want to know what the aliens look like, how they behave, and what they know about the universe. We've never had anyone say to us: "Let's go out and kill the aliens and eat them."

Humankind's first tentative steps to go out and actively search for life on other planets has been marked by immense respect for life too.

When the Galileo spacecraft to Jupiter ended its useful life, NASA controllers dispatched it to its doom in the intense heat of the giant planet's interior, rather than risking it colliding with the icy moon Europa—and potentially contaminating any indigenous life there.

Space agencies from all countries have taken huge care to avoid contamination of Mars, the planet where life is most likely.

"A spacecraft may look gleamingly clean when it's built," says John Rummel—who used to be NASA's splendidly titled planetary protection officer—"but it may harbor over 100 million microbes. We aim to reduce that bio-load down to 300,000 microbes—or even down to 30,000."

By measures like this, we are trying to make sure that our space missions to Mars are not inadvertently weapons of biological warfare—laden with terrestrial bugs that may kill or consume any indigenous Martian life.

And when humans land, the mission planners are determined they will respect Martian microbes, too. NASA engineer Jerry Sanders tells us that the issue has already come up at a meeting to discuss how humans would extract and sterilize Martian water for drinking. He put the following scenario to the team: "OK, you've drilled, you've found water, you've found life—now can I run it through an electrolyzer and kill it?"

After an initial burst of laughter, he tells us, everyone became very thoughtful. A colleague said, "Until you find the next pool of water that has life in it, you can't touch the first one!"

Scientists are respecting the life of another world, however lowly it may be.

Mars teaches us another lesson, too. Space agencies and private organizations are racing to put the first colonies on the planet's red desert. These pioneer astronauts can't take all their food from

Earth—the payload would be just too massive. Instead, they will have to live off the land, farming crop plants within pressurized greenhouses.

And no one envisages taking farm animals to Mars, to raise and slaughter them for food. It would be a waste of the colonists' precious resources: water and the vegetable foodstuff that humans could eat directly.

Bas Lansdorp, CEO of Mars One, an initiative to send settlers on a one-way-trip to the Red Planet, has told us directly: "Plants will grow in Martian gravity, and our colonists will grow all their own food from the start." Having to be vegetarian for the rest of their lives didn't stop over 200,000 people applying for the Mars One mission.

Leading entrepreneur Elon Musk, who founded the rocket company SpaceX, has plans for a city of up to 80,000 people on Mars. Again they would have to be vegetarian; or, strictly speaking, vegan—as there won't be any animal products such as milk or eggs.

The China space agency has built a greenhouse in Beijing to study plants that could provide food and oxygen for future expeditions living on Mars. And NASA has even drawn up a list of the best crops to grow on the Red Planet. How's this for your future menu?— tomatoes, lettuce, radishes, peppers, spring onions, spinach, carrots, cabbage, and herbs, followed by strawberries for dessert.

The cosmic perspective, we believe, should teach us important lessons about what we eat here on planet Earth. When we travel to another world, we will not object to a nonmeat diet. And everyone we've spoken to—scientists and the general public alike—is unequivocal that we should respect any life that we find elsewhere in the universe, be it great or small.

We urge that the same consideration be extended to advanced forms of life on the one world in the whole cosmos where we know that living creatures actually exist—planet Earth.

GLOBAL MEGA-TRENDS AND THE ROLE OF THE FOOD BUSINESS

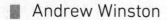 Andrew Winston

Author of *The Big Pivot*

We humans are facing unprecedented challenges as we move deeper into the twenty-first century. Consider a few of the largest mega-forces: climate change and extreme weather, resource constraints and volatile prices for the key inputs to our economy and society (food, energy, metals, and so on), and a level of technology-enabled transparency that allows us to ask new questions about the products we use and the companies that make them. These mega-trends are changing how we live our lives and are pushing the business world in particular to fundamentally change how it operates.

At the center of all three big trends sits the thing we consume most frequently: food. A changing climate and stressed global resource pool (particularly in regard to water) has profoundly impacted our food system. At the same time, transparency is changing our expectations about what we put in our bodies. We're asking new, pressing questions about what's in our food, what it takes to grow and produce that food, and how much of this material we are wasting. Perhaps the most basic question of all, however, is how much meat are we each choosing to consume.

Individual dietary choices are both personal and cultural, of course, but the collective impact of billions of decisions has very real implications for how the entire world evolves. The way we answer all these big questions will largely determine whether the 9 billion people that will soon share this planet will be able to thrive equally.

The way we think about food is a critically important aspect of climate change, the most fundamental and complicated challenge the human race has ever faced. In total the agriculture industry accounts for about 30 percent of the carbon emissions on the planet. This number includes the energy needed to produce food, but also the carbon released while mowing down trees for cattle or farmland (which in large part goes to feed livestock anyway). Our most pressing and precious resource challenge, the availability of clean water, also relies largely on the choices we make about food. The food and agriculture industry is the dominant user of water—up to 70 percent of all water withdrawals.

So food is intricately wrapped up in the two big mega-trends of climate change and resource availability. Agriculture's enormous and outsize impact will, one hopes, put pressure on the food industry to find ways to improve. But the third mega-trend, increased transparency, may be having the greatest impact on our food system. Consumers and businesses now demand more information about the food they buy. While mandatory nutrition labels started the conversation years ago, new demands are changing the food business today faster than ever before.

In the past few years alone, many of the world's largest food companies have announced major shifts in their approach to ingredients and production transparency. McDonald's is implementing new sustainable beef policies and will only buy chicken raised without the antibiotics that are important to human medicine. Tyson Foods, the largest poultry producer in the United States, is eliminating those same antibiotics. General Mills is reducing genetically modified organisms and sugar in its products. Kraft, Taco Bell, Pizza Hut, and Subway are among the many chains announcing drastic reductions in their use of artificial colors and preservatives.

These moves are part of a larger shift toward a so-called clean label approach to food and personal care products: a commitment to reducing the total number of ingredients, using foods that are recognizable as food (that is, avoiding long chemical names), and sourcing food that's as natural as possible (although defining *natural* is trickier than many people realize).

Companies are taking these complicated and sometimes expensive steps because people want to know what exactly they are eating and increasingly expect that information to be easily available. (Note: In some cases the government has officially mandated the information be readily available.) With this increased transparency, it's no surprise companies are trying to clean up their act. If you have to be naked, you might as well look good doing it.

So will this movement toward cleaner, simpler foods impact how much meat we all eat? Perhaps, but it's hard to say. There is clearly a desire for more naturally raised beef, pork, poultry, and fish. And the number of people experimenting with reducetarian-type commitments to eat less meat—either for a day, a week, or for certain parts of the day—is rising.

At the same time, however, the growth of the global middle class is driving increased consumption of meat, particularly pork (half the pigs in the world are in China). There are clearly competing forces at work. But ultimately the largest issues—climate change and resource constraints—will trump all others. Resource-intensive products, be they energy-hogging vehicles or actual hogs, will become more expensive than other options either through reduced availability or commonsense regulation. After all, nothing shifts behavior more efficiently than economics.

For now, food businesses and restaurants will continue to react to market dynamics like shifting input costs: As food prices rose in the first half of this decade, for example, value meals and dollar menus became harder to maintain. Rising costs of production will drive change, but so will shifting preferences. In the fast-food world, companies have attempted to introduce vegetarian and healthier options for years, and there have been (very) few success stories. In Sweden, for example, the midsize chain Max Burgers has for years pushed healthier options and encouraged consumers to reduce their carbon footprint by eating less meat. The chain has since experienced encouragingly high profit margins.

Unfortunately, vegetarian and healthful options at the biggest brands have had more mixed results, making companies wary of taking big risks. And yet, chains like Panera and Chipotle have demonstrated there's strong demand for healthier foods with cleaner labels. Chipotle has had significant success with its overall pitch about sourcing (grass-fed beef, for example) and has done well with its sofritas (a tofu-based filling for burritos)—40 percent of customers who buy this vegan option are not vegetarians. With a quarter of U.S. adults now saying they are reducing meat to some extent, companies will take notice.

The food business, our eating habits, and the earth are all chang-ing in important ways, and these shifts are reinforcing each other. In the near future, the world of food will look much different from how it does today, and it will certainly include less mass-produced meat.

FEEDING THE WORLD AND MAKING ROOM FOR ALL SPECIES

Emma Marris

Author of *Rambunctious Garden: Saving Nature in a Post-Wild World*

The western prairie fringed orchid (*Platanthera praeclara*) is a stun-ning spring flower of the tallgrass prairie. Each stalk is up to two feet tall and covered in dozens of elaborately fringed white flowers. It is also threatened with extinction because only tiny scraps of tallgrass prairie remain in North America. About 96 percent of this once vast and diverse landscape has been plowed under. Corn and soy grow there now, in neat rows. Who eats all this corn and soy? Not us.

In fact, 36 percent of crops around the world are used to feed livestock. In the United States, the figure is 57 percent.[1] The num-ber one threat to endangered species is habitat loss. The number one cause of habitat loss is agricultural expansion. And by far the least efficient use of agricultural land is meat production.

When people eat plants, most of the energy in the crops ends up in people's bellies. But when people eat animals, which in turn ate plants, a mere 12 percent of the energy of the crops ends up in peo-ple's bellies. The rest is lost. That means we can feed more people with the same amount of land if we all eat less meat. And that's even before accounting for the vast areas of the Earth used as pasture land.

Beef cattle, in particular, are enormous users of land. Mind bogglingly, they use 160 times as much land per calorie as rice, potatoes, or wheat.[2] Producing poultry, pork, eggs, and dairy also requires a significant amount of land, on average six times as much as the three plant staples.

This huge land use is a direct threat to the western prairie fringed orchid and hundreds of other species that are endangered because of habitat conversion to agriculture, which has already mowed over 70 percent of the world's grassland, 50 percent of its savanna, 45 percent of its temperate deciduous forest, and 27 percent of its tropical forest.[3] And as the global population grows—and gets richer and potentially eager to eat more meat—agriculture expansion could drive species extinct, erase whole ecosystem types, and convert our world to an endless expanse of dull monocultures. All this land clearing and agriculture are also massive contributors to climate change as forests are burned and livestock release methane.

When faced with the challenge of an expanding and increasingly affluent global human population, the knee-jerk response has been to think about ways we can grow more food on more land. But that is not the only path forward. We can feed the world now and in the future without expanding lands devoted to agriculture.

In 2011, a diverse group of environmental and agricultural scholars wrote a paper in the scientific journal *Nature* in which they explained how. First, we can use tried-and-true technologies to improve how much food can be grown on each acre—that is, to improve yield. In poorer parts of the world, yields are much lower than in Europe and the United States. This yield gap could be closed using a mix of techniques from organic farming and "precision farming," by which GPS and satellite imagery helps farmers add just enough water and fertilizer to each plant rather than bathing the whole field in excess water and chemicals. Better seed varieties and breeding higher-yielding varieties of so-called orphan crops like yams, groundnuts, tef, and cassava can help too.

Second, we must attack food waste at all points on the chain between farm and compost heap. A shocking one third of the food we grow is never eaten.

Third, we must cut back on growing crops for biofuel and to feed to animals. The group estimated that if sixteen major crops were eaten instead of fed to cars, trucks, cows, pigs, chickens, and other meat animals, we would have a billion more tons of food every year—a 49 percent increase in calories. That's huge. At that rate, we could do more than stop agricultural expansion. We could give some land back to the species with which we share the planet. We could reseed grasslands and come back to listen to the meadowlarks sing. We could watch the tropical forest regrow and the orangutans fan out into new homelands. We could watch African wild dogs romp on expanded savanna.

A key point here is that we don't have to all become vegans to make profound changes in our agricultural systems. As the authors of the *Nature* paper write, "While wholesale conversions of the human diet and the elimination of food waste are not realistic goals, even incremental steps could be extremely beneficial."

Today, people in China, India, and Southeast Asia eat diets heavy on plants and light on meat. But they are getting richer. Will they maintain those plant-based diets or switch over to the hamburgers and chicken patties of North America? And will we keep eating all those hamburgers and chicken patties once we see how much land it takes?

While governments can use taxes and incentives to try to shift citizens' diets, it may be the cumulative weight of billions of individual decisions that will allow humans to feed ourselves without driving countless other species extinct. Reducing our poultry, beef, and pork consumption can have a real positive effect if enough of us do it. And on an individual level, cutting back on meat can be a powerful way of enacting your own belief that other species have a right to continued existence on Earth and that the planet is not ours to turn into a giant spherical feedlot.

I eat meat. But I am happy to eat it much less frequently if it means that there will be western prairie fringed orchids in the world.

IT'S ABOUT MUCH MORE THAN MEAT

▌ Joan Dye Gussow

Mary Swartz Rose Professor Emerita and former chair, Nutrition Education Program, Teachers College, Columbia University, and author of *Growing, Older: A Chronicle of Death, Life, and Vegetables*

"Meatless." In the United States, the operative word for a meal prepared entirely with vegetable matter is not a joyous invitation to what's on the plate—"crunchy," "rich," "spicy," or even "light"—but what's not there: the meal is "meatless." Although meat consumption appears to be suffering a moment of slightly waning popularity, our national eaters have for centuries been serious consumers of animal flesh.

Although the earliest settlers were accomplished as neither fisherfolk nor hunters, fish, shellfish and game were so abundant on this rich continent that they almost asked to be eaten. "The diet of the seventeenth century was indeed dominated by game," food historians Waverly Root and Richard de Rochemont wrote, "that of the eighteenth leaned heavily upon it, and it remained important in the nineteenth up to the Civil War. . . . For a considerable time after the arrival of the first settlers, game was not only the main meat of the colonists, it was often the main food." So meat eating was our national norm, and we regularly ate enough of it to be the envy of the people we left behind. When the Irish immigrants wrote letters home saying they ate meat every day, their relatives wrote back in disbelief.

And now? "Every day" is putting it modestly, "every meal" is more like it. The Web site of the seriously conservationist David Suzuki Foundation currently recommends: "Try to eat at least one meat-free meal per day."

Something over 100 years ago each of us annually ate a little over 100 pounds of flesh, about half of it beef. Four decades later, it was pork Spammed for the troops that spiked World War II meat consumption, and after the war, steaks on the backyard grill and McDonald's burgers pushed beef to its 1976 high of almost 89 pounds a year for each of us, pushing the total flesh on our plates to the then record of 138 pounds. At that point, beef consumption began declining, by roughly 10 pounds a decade.

But thanks to the buckets and breasts of chicken we increasingly brought to our tables, poultry consumption climbed during those years at almost the same rate, pushing our flesh consumption to its 2004 peak of just over 170 pounds.

In short, we're persistent meat eaters, and a recent slight decline in consumption likely reflects a depressed supply, not a change in our tastes. Although figures vary by source, only 2 to 3+ percent of American adults are currently flesh abstainers, 10 percent have been vegetarian or vegan at one time or another, and a *Vegetarian Times* study found that a mere 5.2 percent were "definitely interested" in trying such a diet in the future.

Given the obvious stubbornness of our meat habit, what will it take to move people to leave half of the flesh off their plates? I used to think just calling it "flesh" would help make eating meat less attractive, like calling fat "grease," but grossness is too ordinary now to provoke a diet change.

One would like to believe that simple pleas for compassion could win over even serious consumers, but the brutalities of confined animal feeding operations (CAFOs) are increasingly familiar and, like the repeated efforts in print and on film to make us see flesh on the table as dead animals, seem to have had little obvious impact on how much of those animals we all eat. People don't want to know how their red or white meat got into those plastic packages, and telling them clearly doesn't turn most of them toward flesh-free meals. Indeed, several years ago the *New York Times* ran an op-ed piece actually suggesting that because CAFOs were here to stay, we could genetically engineer animals to suffer less in their hellholes.

There are lots of other ideas out there. You can teach people how to enjoy vegetable matter by having them over for dinner, failing to announce that the meal is meat free. I remember a guest of mine remarking, as she savored pasta rich with a meatless tomato sauce, how difficult it was to plan a meal for a vegetarian. On a larger scale, we could make feeding oneself without meat a mandatory survival skill to be taught in school so coming generations could learn how to prepare plant-based meals that are quick, easy, and delicious. And we could make our public efforts more positive: Vegetable Garden Tuesdays might seem more appealing than Meatless Mondays.

And because people are eating out so much, we need to convince ordinary eateries—not just gourmet dining spots—to make a vegetarian option the daily special from time to time. And to make their standard portion sizes of meat smaller—I was recently served an eight-ounce hamburger as if it were normal—which would also help solve our obesity problem. And of course it would be useful to ban "all you can eat" advertising. As long as the meat lobby has the clout to buy off legislators, however, rational national dietary guidance that might reduce our flesh consumption will be blocked by Congress.

But in the end, convincing people to reduce their meat consumption is probably not the task we need to undertake. Not that it wouldn't help to eat less beef, given the amount of grain, forage, water, land, and energy it takes to make each quarter-pound burger, but we could all stop eating meat tomorrow and if we kept devouring the rest of the world's resources at our present rate, we would still be driving fast toward disaster.

Because the issue really isn't meat, but lack of mindfulness about our impact on the planet. Our national extravagance in regard to meat—our on-average consumption of twice as much as we need—is merely a single example of our national overconsumption of everything. And it's everything—our throw-away cheap clothes, our rapidly outdated (and replaced!) electronics, our bloated vehicles, our mansions—that's going to kill us in the end.

So just as the papal encyclical wasn't really about planetary warming but about the cruel global fall-outs from the century or so that us rich folks have devoted to devouring the planet, our meat problem is simply part of our mindless consumption, part of our throwaway culture, as *Laudato si'* puts it, of "compulsive consumerism" that "quickly reduces things to rubbish."

Whenever we buy something, anything, we are investing in our planet's future. If it is a material object, someone somewhere made it, and the wood or metal or fiber or soil or water it took to produce it came from somewhere, and your purchase either contributed to making that someone's life tolerable or not and to sustaining the planet's web of life or not. We're well overdue to pay attention and stop devouring a lot more than meat.

INSECTS. THEY'RE WHAT'S FOR DINNER.

▌ Daniella Martin

Author of *Edible: An Adventure into the World of Eating Insects and the Last Great Hope to Save the Planet*

When I first began promoting insects as a sustainable protein source, I was often met with astonishment and confusion. Lately when the topic comes up, however, the reaction is much more open. It's clear that entomophagy is spreading.

While perhaps unconventional in the West, insects have long stood out as a sustainable protein source, especially when measured against other popular meat. For one thing, they are cold-blooded. In contrast to cows, who spend a huge amount of their energy heating their bodies, insects don't spend a nutritional cent on body heat. All of their energy goes toward two things: growth and reproduction.

A female cricket has a lifespan of three months. During that time, she will lay around 100 eggs. Being conservative, let's say that just twenty-five of those eggs become viable female crickets who in turn lay 100 eggs. Again being conservative, let's say one quarter of the resulting 2,500 eggs hatch viable females. Within months, your potential cricket population is up to 60,000—and that's starting from one fertilized female. Edible cricket farms I have visited in Thailand had dozens of cricket pens, all open to the air, smelling faintly of corn feed and sounding like a sleigh bell factory.

For all of this reproductive potential, crickets require very little space, making them ideal for urban farming. Keeping production close to consumption means less energy spent on transportation. Also, edible insects generally require very little processing. An incredible amount of resources, both human and natural, go into processing meat, from the slaughtering and cleaning to the butchering and packing. For example, up to 40 percent of a chicken doesn't wind up on our plates. Meanwhile, a cricket is typically eaten whole. The frozen foods section of Thailand's version of Costco sells one-pound bags of whole crickets. In the United States, crickets are typically cooked, dried, and then ground into flour, a process so simple it could be done in an apartment kitchen.

Partly because they are consumed whole, insects are excellent sources of nutrition. High in protein, essential fatty acids, iron, calcium, B_{12}, zinc, and other nutrients, insects are in many ways an ideal food source. While they may seem new and exotic to us, our ancestors relied on them for millennia. Even generally herbivorous gorillas have been known to eat bugs when it's convenient.

With so many clear benefits, why is there still such a mental block against using insects as food? Many people are afraid they will taste bad. After all, insects are typically depicted as what I like to call the Three D's: dirty, diseased, and disgusting. Cockroaches, for instance, are associated mainly with squalid conditions and the spread of disease. In reality, only a handful of the over 4,000 species of cockroach have any connection to humans. Vivid blue, green, and iridescent cockroaches exist in jungles around the world, far from our apartment sinks.

To prove that our insect squeamishness is mostly psychological, I invited a group of 100 people to taste three dishes while blindfolded. Two of the dishes, I told them, contained insects. Their job was to figure out which of the three dishes was bug free. The trick, of course, was that all three dishes contained bugs.

I wasn't surprised to find that people had a hard time deciding which dish tasted bug free. Some thought it was the cricket granola, which happened to contain whole crickets. Others were sure it was the mealworm Rice Krispy treats, which was chock-full of whole mealworms. Most people were convinced it was the cricket-powder-based Chirp Chips. When I revealed the truth, the surprise in the room was palpable (pun intended—palpi are the appendages insects use to taste).

Although still a few steps ahead of its time, the idea of eating insects is steadily creeping into the mainstream. Health food stores around the country have begun carrying bug-based protein bars. As recently as a few years ago, if you wanted to try cricket flour cookies, you had to order the crickets live from what was essentially a bait farm. They'd arrive, still chirping, in a box at your front door and you'd have to freeze them overnight before roasting and eventually grinding them up into flour. Obviously, this process isn't for everyone. Luckily, today all you have to do is order the finely milled, organic, human-grade bug flour online.

Expanding our collective palates to include insects could help reduce the amount of natural resources used to produce conventional animal protein. And with the human population expected to hit 9 billion by 2050, experts say we'll need to increase food production by 50 percent. Insects could go a long way toward ensuring we are able to meet that mark.

MAKING THE INVISIBLE VISIBLE: EXPLOITATION OF LIVESTOCK WORKERS SUPPORTS THE MEAT INDUSTRY

Molly Anderson

William R. Kenan Professor of food studies, Middlebury College

Livestock production in the United States relies on a legion of low-paid workers, most coming from Mexico in search of jobs, and about half without documentation. The arduous pilgrimage from their homes to farms and ranches in the United States is part of the story of meat, and the meat industry would not be able to sell meat at current prices without exploiting these workers. This essay explores the connections among the meat industry, workers' well-being, and meat consumption.

The most recent figures on farm labor from the National Agricultural Statistic Service's Farm Labor Survey indicate that 872,000 farmworkers were employed on U.S. crop and livestock farms in mid-July of 2015. The Department of Labor's National Agricultural Workers Survey showed that 71 percent of crop workers surveyed between 2007 and 2009 were foreign born (with 67 percent from Mexico) and 48 percent were not legally authorized to work in the United States. Comparable figures for livestock workers are not available.

Increasing numbers of migrants came to the United States from Mexico since the North American Free Trade Area of the Americas (NAFTA) agreement was signed into law on January 1, 1994, opening a floodgate of cheap corn and other commodities from the United States to Mexico. Mexican farmers could no longer sell their crops on the market because the cost of subsidized crops from the United

States was below the cost of production in Mexico. Thousands of former farmers migrated north in search of jobs that could provide a decent income for their families. Migrants have poured into rural Southeastern and Southwestern states in particular, and many of them end up in meat processing, dairy production, and chicken or pork confined animal feeding operations (CAFOs). These industries went through a major restructuring between the 1980s and early 2000s, moving from the Midwest to Southern states and becoming concentrated under just a few brands.

In search of jobs and trying to escape deportation to their home countries, workers land all over the United States. They have almost no control over working conditions and wages, which are often deplorable. Farm wages vary significantly by task, industry, region, and legal status, but on average, farmworkers have among the lowest annual earnings of all U.S. workers, both because their hourly wages are relatively low and because many farmworkers are unable to find year-round employment in agriculture. The latest data from the National Agricultural Statistics Service indicates that livestock workers were paid on average $12.02/hour during mid-October. Between 1990 and 2012, the average real hourly wage of hired farmworkers who were not in supervisory positions (including both documented and undocumented workers) increased by 19 percent, reaching $10.80 per hour in 2012. This increase was not large enough to narrow the average gap between farm and nonfarm wages. Farm wages have typically been about half the average wage of nonfarm workers and about one dollar per hour less than wages in the "leisure and hospitality" sector, another low-wage industry that depends heavily on foreign-born workers.

Surveys of working conditions in different parts of the United States over the past decade have repeatedly found human rights abuses, substandard wages, and abysmal housing and working conditions in the meat-production and -processing industries. Human Rights Watch published *Blood, Sweat, and Fear: Workers' Rights in U.S. Meat and Poultry Plants* in 2004. This was followed in 2009 by Nebraska Appleseed's report, *The Speed Kills You: The Voice of Nebraska's Meatpacking Workers*. Both reports documented serious abuse, including inhumane line-speeds in meat-packing plants, where workers were expected to process up to 400 head of livestock per hour with electric knives while standing in the cold on slippery floors. Sexual and ethnic harassment, verbal and emotional abuse, lack of information about workers' compensation, and restrictions on the freedom to organize were commonly reported. In 2014, Migrant Justice found through a survey of 172 dairy workers in Vermont that 40 percent earned less than Vermont's minimum wage of $9/hour, 40 percent had no time off, 29 percent work seven or more hours without a break to eat, 20 percent had their first paycheck illegally withheld, and 30 percent had experienced a workplace injury or illness. In a survey conducted between 2013 and 2015, Oxfam America found low wages, scant benefits, workers fired for speaking up or complaining, and high rates of injury and illness in poultry-processing plants in Southeastern states.

In addition to poor working conditions and wages, workers in the meat industry face unique health risks. Many diseases are transmitted between humans and livestock, including strains of influenza and tuberculosis. The dust in CAFOs can set off asthma attacks, and gases from manure, such as ammonia, are harmful to respiratory health. One of the most serious health impacts of work in livestock operations has only recently been brought to light: growing incidence of antibiotic resistance (ABR) due to the practice of adding low doses of common antibiotics to the feed (subtherapeutic doses). Bacteria mutate into resistant strains and become prevalent in the soil and feeding area. Therefore, simple infections that previously could be treated with common antibiotics such as penicillin, streptomycin, or erythromycin are resistant even to combinations of antibiotics. While ABR can affect anyone, workers in industrialized meat production facilities are exposed to the highest concentrations and newest mutations.

The most promising improvements in conditions for workers in meat production and processing have come about through farmworker organizing. Despite having little power vis-à-vis managers and the corporations that control the meat industry, workers have initiated several successful campaigns. Two notable campaigns are Milk with Dignity in Vermont, modeled after the very successful strategies of the Coalition of Immokalee Workers, and a new effort to benefit workers in chicken-processing factories supported by Oxfam America. Milk with Dignity was organized by Migrant Justice, and targets Ben & Jerry's. Their goals include dignified work and quality housing, freedom of movement and access to transportation, freedom from discrimination, and access to healthcare. Among their accomplishments are passage of legislation in Vermont to prohibit state police from using public resources for deportation, extending the right to get a driver's license to all residents of the state regardless of immigration status, including undocumented workers in universal healthcare coverage, and expanding state power to collect unpaid wages.

Could reducing meat consumption also help workers in the meat industry? In the short term, this is not likely. With less demand for the products from meat-producing farms, their workers would be forced to find other employment, possibly at lower wages. But if the only farms selling meat were ones that guaranteed fair wages and good working conditions for employees, and if reduced consumption were linked to worker exploitation (for example, through a boycott), and if stockholders demanded that publicly owned companies buy only from farms certified to have good conditions, then farms that currently treat workers badly would be encouraged to improve working conditions and wages.

Many farmers insist that they want to treat workers well but cannot afford to make improvements in housing or to pay more. Charging more for meat, to compensate for paying workers better, may make meat inaccessible to many consumers. This would result in lower consumption de facto, although through a policy that affects low-income consumers disproportionately. For real solutions to the labor problems in the meat industry, workers need far more than voluntary measures by benevolent farmers. At a minimum, fixing the broken migration system into the United States is necessary so that workers can freely travel to and from jobs and seek employment at the farms that provide the best wages and working conditions.

HELP SAVE THE PLANET: TAKE THE ½ CO$_2$E CHALLENGE!

■ Oscar E. Fernandez

Author of *Everyday Calculus: Discovering the Hidden Math All Around Us*

You probably think about the health implications of your diet often—many of us do. What you may not think about is the implications your food choices have for the *planet's* health. I'm not here to guilt-trip you into being a vegetarian—this is, after all, a book about *reduce*tarian solutions. Instead, I'd like to help you understand how your food choices contribute to global greenhouse gas emissions (GHGEs), and then challenge you to cut your food-related GHGE in half. And I'll help you do it.

Let's start with the data. In 2011, the Environmental Working Group (EWG)—a nonprofit environmental research organization based in Washington, D.C.—published the results of a comprehensive study of GHGE organized by food category. Titled "Meat Eater's Guide to Climate Change + Health," the study draws on several data sources (including peer-reviewed journal articles, reports from the UN's Intragovernmental Panel on Climate Change, and publications from several U.S. government agencies) to estimate the cradle-to-grave kilograms (kg) of the carbon dioxide equivalent (CO_2e) of GHGEs for various foods. These emissions result from the production and postproduction activities (including transportation) required to deliver 1 kg of a particular food. Animal products, in particular meat, dominate the top of the list: lamb comes in first (39.2 kg CO_2e per kg), followed by beef (27 kg CO_2e per kg), cheese (13.5 kg CO_2e per kg), and pork (12.1 kg CO_2e per kg). But because we're not used to thinking of our diet in terms of how many *kilograms* of food we eat, let's convert the Environmental Working Group's numbers to kilograms of CO_2e per *food calorie*.

The first step is to divide EWG's numbers by 10 to get kilograms of CO_2e per 100 grams of food. Then, we divide the result by the number of calories in a 100-gram serving of whatever food we're calculating for. This will give us an idea of the amount of emissions produced per calorie. For example, according to Google a 100-gram serving of 85 percent lean ground beef contains 250 calories, so 1 calorie of this lean beef requires $27 \div 10 \div 250 = 0.0108$ kg of CO_2e emissions to get to your plate. That's a tiny number! Let's make things easier by multiplying by 1,000 to convert to grams of CO_2e emissions per calorie (arriving at 10.8 g CO_2e per calorie of beef, for example). With all of EWG's numbers converted to grams of CO_2e per calorie, we can now calculate the food-related GHGEs of an entire diet.

Let's suppose that, as a percentage of your daily calories, your diet consists of: b percent beef, c percent chicken, d percent dairy, g percent grains, l percent legumes, and v percent vegetables. Using the mathematical steps just outlined, your diet's "carbon intensity"—the grams of CO_2e per calorie associated with your diet—is approximately:

$$CID = 10.8b + 4.2c + 3.5d + 2g + 0.5l + 4.8v$$

(*Note*: CID in this equation stands for carbon intensity of the diet.) To make the calculation easier I've created a free, customizable CID calculator on my Web site: surroundedbymath.com/interactive -math. But let's do another calculation by hand just for extra. Consider a hypothetical diet that's 10 percent beef, 10 percent chicken, 15 percent dairy, 40 percent grains, 5 percent legumes, and 20 percent vegetables. Then:

$$CID = 10.8(0.10) + 4.2(0.10) + 3.5(0.15) + 2(0.4) + 0.5(0.05) + 4.8(0.2)$$

This translates to 3.81 grams CO_2e per calorie. When adjusted for a 2,000 calorie daily intake, this diet will require 7,620 grams (7.62 kg) of CO_2e emissions. That's equivalent to burning 7.3 pounds of coal—and that's only for one day and one person. Cue my ½ CO_2e challenge.

I know what you're thinking: "How in the world am I going to cut my CID number in half?" It's going to take a lot of determination—and a little bit of math as well. Suppose we swapped 1 percent of our hypothetical diet's beef calories for legumes, so that "b" decreases by 1 while "l" increases by 1. The decrease in b lowers CID by 10.8(0.01) = 0.108, while the increase in l raises CID by 0.5(0.01) = 0.005. The net effect is a CID number that's lower by 0.103. That would lower the CID of the hypothetical diet to 3.81 – 0.103 = 3.707, which is about 2.7 percent lower. Now we've discovered that the coefficients of the variables in the CID equation tell us how much the CID will increase or decrease when the caloric intake of each food group is increased or decreased by 1 percent. Beef has the largest coefficient and legumes the smallest, so you get the biggest reduction in CID by swapping beef for legume calories. (Black bean burgers, here we come!) More generally, because I've calculated that the coefficients for lamb, turkey, and farmed salmon all turn out to be at least 9 (see the aforementioned Web site if you're curious about my methodology), the math clearly shows that the best way to lower your diet's carbon intensity is by eating less animal meat, be that red meat, poultry, or seafood (and, ideally, swapping those calories for legume calories).

I hope you now see how useful the CID equation is. Sure, it's only an estimate of a diet's carbon footprint. But the beef coefficient's outsize influence is a clear indicator of the scale to which different food choices impact the environment. This isn't speculation anymore; it's arithmetic. That's why I hope you'll join the Reducetarian movement. You'll be reducing your carbon footprint, and assuming you swap those meat-heavy calories for healthful foods, you're probably adopting a healthier lifestyle as a bonus. So take the ½ CO_2e challenge—your body, your math teachers, and your planet will thank you.

THE FOOD DESERT PHENOMENON

■ Hillary Shaw

Author of *The Consuming Geographies of Food: Diet, Food Deserts and Obesity*

The term *food desert* was first coined in Glasgow, Scotland, in 1996 to describe the absence of local retailers selling affordable healthy food in poverty-stricken neighborhoods.[1] However, studies looking at the lack of physical access to local food retailing in English villages had been conducted by the Women's Institute as early as the 1970s. At that time, widows without cars had become isolated; local food stores were closing down, and a decline in bus services made transportation almost impossible without a car. By 2000, food deserts had been discovered in several British cities, including Coventry, where they were described as "areas where cheap nutritious food is virtually unobtainable. Car-less residents . . . depend on the corner shop where prices are high and fresh produce is poor or non-existent." Worse, many residents were becoming reliant on nutritionally deficient takeout restaurants.

Several technological, socioeconomic and political processes came together to create the food desert phenomenon. For one thing, personal transport shifted to cars, leaving behind those unable to drive. At the same time, food retailing was being transformed by economies of scale, with supermarkets and their cheaper prices causing many small independent shops to close. A local food store requires a customer pool of a few hundred people whereas a large superstore requires some 10,000 consumers. In the middle are typical UK discount stores, like Co-operative or Tesco Express, which require 2,000 or 3,000 customers. This means the opening of one supermarket can cause the closure of twenty local shops, denuding several square kilometers of all food retailing, with the exception of fast food.

Meanwhile, these developments were themselves products of a shift, in the late 1970s, away from Fordist accumulative capitalism toward a globalized neo-liberal model that greatly increased inequality within developed countries. This shift also precipitated a more vocational approach to education, as UK schools in the 1980s dropped cooking lessons in favor of science and mathematics. As a result, a whole generation grew up without culinary skills. The spread of microwave ovens and ready meals, which undermined local greengrocers and butchers, solidified an attitude of "food as fuel."

There are three levels of (impeded) access that create food deserts: poor physical access to retailers; poor financial access as household food budgets shrink; and poor information access as the skills required to prepare a healthy meal from raw ingredients wither away. Other societal changes only exacerbate these trends. Social ties have weakened, reducing help for shoppers who might be elderly or infirm. Meanwhile, increased traffic and crime have closed many smaller shops and made others hard to reach. The arrival of the Internet and increasing time pressures at home have shifted preferences toward unhealthy, ready-to-eat meals while removing incentives to cook. The only thing we don't demand from food is that it be healthful—for us or the environment.

The irony is nobody starves in a food desert; food is plentiful but not nutritious. Inhabitants overconsume calorific food but miss out on vitamins. Cheap, fatty, sugary food is cheaper than healthy food, a phenomenon called the "health premium." This gap widened between 1989 and 2007 in Britain and is even larger in less affluent areas where a basket of healthy food costs 58 percent more than obesogenic cheap meats and sugary fare. As a Birmingham nutritionist recently told me, "Burgers are ridiculously cheap round here," highlighting the lack of financial incentive to eat healthy. Any fresh produce stocked by independent shopkeepers in food desert areas is likely to spoil before it can be sold, eroding already-low profit levels. Such shops therefore tend to stock only "hard," longer-lasting vegetables such as potatoes, carrots, and turnips. A councilor for Halton Moor, a lower-income part of Leeds, noted casually the area's malnourished children. It was almost as if this was natural, that malnourishment was to be expected despite being within sight of the prosperous city center.

Meat is cheap because free-market production and trade doesn't have to allow for externalities such as health or the environment. Just as Nauru islanders have a high obesity rate because they eat fatty "flap meat," deprived consumers in European and U.S. food deserts are becoming obese in part due to mass-produced beef burgers and cheap sugary foodstuffs. The real retail price of sugar, £300 a kilo in the year 1400, fell to under £10 in the 1800s and is now below £1. We need to reconnect the poor with healthy inexpensive food, perhaps locally produced through projects such as urban farms, allotments, or a modern Dig for Victory program. Demand for fresh produce could be stimulated through healthy eating leaflets and cookery classes hosted at job and community centers in food desert areas.

The costs of such a food reconnection program would be more than recouped through a reduction in the costs of obesity-induced illnesses. The UK's National Health Service spends some £10 billion annually on such illnesses, but the total cost to Britain is nearer £25 billion. The issue of course is time. Just as consumers in food deserts fuel up on cheap meat and sugar, giving little thought to future health consequences, so too are governments unwilling to spend money on initiatives that won't pay dividends until the future. The pertinent question becomes how long can we afford *not* to preserve both our own health and that of the planet? What we do to tackle the food desert phenomenon is a kind of litmus test—and the future depends on how willing we are to act.

THE GLOBAL MAP OF WHO EATS TOO MUCH MEAT

▉ Benjamin Hennig

Assistant professor in geography, University of Iceland

▉ Danny Dorling

Author of *Inequality and the 1%*

International data on the consumption of red meat, poultry, and seafood is not especially reliable because different sources of data from reputable bodies give very different results. We know that collectively, humanity eats far too much meat and that the amount we are eating, farming, and killing is increasing rapidly. But we shouldn't assume this problem is a universal one. In fact, just a few countries are responsible for almost all of the world's meat consumption.

Before analyzing this global map of meat consumption, it is worth considering just how much meat exists. It is interesting that a great deal of this flesh is—not to be too macabre—made up of humans. When the world population passed 7 billion people in 2011, we humans weighed, in total, 385 million tons. And that number is rising. Humans are already collectively the heaviest animals on the planet—except for the ones we farm for their meat. This includes some 1.4 billion cattle weighing a total of 573 million tons at any one time. Then there are the 1.1 billion sheep—weighing in at 71 million tons—and 18.6 billion chickens—weighing 44 million tons worldwide and by far the most populous birds on the planet today.[1] If we ignore the fish in the oceans and the insects, then the vast majority of animal life on earth, by weight, is either us, or the animals bred specifically to feed us.

Returning to our central topic, there is a huge variation in meat consumption in the affluent developed world today. Let's consider countries of the world ranked by how much meat (kilograms per capita per year) is consumed each year. (Note: these totals exclude fish.) The top five include New Zealand (126.90 kg/capita/year), Australia (121.10 kg/capita/year), the United States (117.60 kg/capita/year), Austria (106.40 kg/capita/year), and Israel (102.00 kg/capita/year).[2]

The maps below summarize these trends and inequalities in global meat consumption. They show meat consumption from three different perspectives. The gray-black shades highlight where the population of a country consumes more meat than the global average. The countries depicted in white consume below the global average.

The top map provides the most conventional perspective using a normal map projection (here, the so-called Robinson projection). The other two maps are cartogram depictions resized according to specific variables: In the first cartogram (the map in the middle), the size of each country is defined by its population. Europe is a densely populated continent and therefore appears bigger, showing the larger impact of the high meat consumption there. Meanwhile countries with above-average meat consumption but smaller populations seem to almost disappear, as is the case with Russia and Canada. Most of the countries with below-average meat consumption—generally in the poorer parts of the world—also stand out because of their large populations.

The third map shows only countries where there is excess meat consumption. Excessive consumption in this context is defined by calculating the global average meat consumption per person compared to a country's average. The difference is then multiplied by the country's population. Countries that consume excessively more meat are shown as proportionally bigger. China, for example, has a much larger population than the United States but shows up as smaller on the map because its meat consumption is lower, on average, than America's.

The point of using these different kinds of cartograms is to show the outsize impact some countries have on our global meat consumption. The wealthy world in particular needs a wake-up call. It's not hopeless, yet. But for the momentum to shift, citizens in affluent, meat-loving nations need to take the first step by collectively reducing the amount of meat that finds its way onto their dining tables.

GLOBAL ABOVE-AVERAGE MEAT CONSUMPTION

CONVENTIONAL MAP
(Robinson projection)

POPULATION CARTOGRAM
(countries resized according to their total population)

EXCESS MEAT CONSUMPTION CARTOGRAM
(countries resized according to their total excess
meat consumption when compared to the global average)

COLOR KEY: Calorie intake from meat, per person compared to global average

- 200% and above
- 150 to under 200%
- 100 to under 150%
- below global average

PERISHING POSSESSIONS

■ Tristram Stuart

Author of *Waste: Uncovering the Global Food Scandal* and
The Bloodless Revolution: A Cultural History of Vegetarian-
ism from 1600 to Modern Times

In the seventeenth century, the English philosopher John Locke argued that if someone took more food than he needed and wasted it, "he took more than his share, and robbed others." If, on the other hand, he consumed, traded, or even gave away his surplus food "he did no injury; he wasted not the common stock; destroyed no part of the portion of goods that belonged to others, so long as nothing perished uselessly in his hands." How do modern wealthy people and nations stand up to Locke's judgments, and do his moral paradigms hold any lessons for us today?

In a globalized food supply chain, the people who depend on the same "common stock" of resources are no longer necessarily our neighbors or even our compatriots. They may live many thousands of miles away: people in Asia and Africa depend on the global marketplace for their food just as do people in Europe and North America. How do we answer for the fact that most countries in Europe and North America waste between a third and half of their total food supplies between the plow and the plate? Whether it is fresh fruit and vegetables rejected by supermarkets for failing to meet arbitrary cosmetic standards or manufacturers forced to discard millions of pounds of meat because they are past their sell-by-date, or whether it is the waste we all witness daily in our own homes—all of this represents land, water, and other resources that could be put to better use than filling garbage dumps with food.

The connection between food profligacy in rich countries and food poverty elsewhere in the world is neither simple nor direct, but it is nevertheless real. Obviously, the solution is not for rich countries to send old sausages or stale bread over to poor countries after saving them from the rubbish bin. This spurious connection assumes that the food in rich people's homes or overstocked super-markets had no other potential destiny than ending up in rich countries in the first place. But there has long been a connection between food being wasted in rich countries and the lack of food on the other side of the world, and the food crisis of 2007–2008 and more recent price spikes, partly caused by global shortages of crops like soy, cereals, and wheat (commonly fed to livestock), has made this even more evident. It is clear that fluctuations in consumption in rich countries affect the availability of food globally, and this directly impacts less wealthy people's ability to buy enough food to survive.

The case for this is easily demonstrated by meat—principally beef, poultry, and seafood—which has global prices determining the cost of food in the markets of Africa and Asia just as it does in the shopping aisles of the United States and Europe. The amount of meat that rich countries import and export depends on how much is used within those countries and how much is thrown away. If Western countries divert millions of pounds of meat into their rub-bish bins, there will be less available on the world market. If they stopped doing so, there would be more, and it would be more likely to be affordable. Because food supply has become a global phenom-enon, and particularly when demand outstrips supply, putting food in the trash really is equivalent to taking it off the world market and out of the mouths of the starving.

Hunger and malnutrition are not exclusively foreign concerns either; millions in the developed world also do not have enough to eat. This situation persists even while supermarkets throw away millions of pounds of quality food.

So in terms of taking food from the mouths of the hungry, how significant is the food wasted in rich countries? One way of looking at this is to calculate the nutritional value of the food being wasted. It is difficult to imagine a million pounds of food, but converting that measurement into the number of people who could have been fed on it makes it more comprehensible, and the value of that food more vivid. It can even help provide a clearer idea of how many people the world would really be able to feed if people cut down on waste.

It is possible to calculate approximately how much food could be saved if all nations in the world reduced waste and unnecessary surplus to the extent that no country supplied its population with more than 130 percent of the population's nutritional needs. At present all wealthy nations in Europe and North America provide their populations with between 150 and 200 percent of their nutritional needs. In other words, their shops and restaurants contain up to twice as much food as is absolutely required. The details of these calculations are laid out more fully in my book *Waste: Uncovering the Global Food Scandal*, but the overall total shows that 33 percent of global food supplies could be saved, or enough food to provide the entire nutritional requirements of an extra 3 billion people.

Even these staggering figures do not include the savings that could be made if Westerners ate a smaller proportion of meat in their diet, which would liberate grains that are inefficiently fed to animals rather than people. Consider that animal protein production requires more than eight times as much fossil-fuel energy as production of plant protein while yielding animal protein that is only marginally more nutritious for humans than the comparable amount of plant protein. More specifically, pigs consume energy in a ratio of approximately 9:1 energy input to protein output; for beef cattle production this ratio is approximately 25:1. Other ratios for turkey, chicken, milk, and eggs are similarly inefficient. With more than a third of global calories and half of global protein inefficiently used as animal feed—the impact of decreasing global meat consumption would be monumental.

It seems that the affluent world is doing on a global scale what Locke warned against in seventeenth-century England. Ultimately it means sequestering the land and other common resources of the world to grow food that is wasted. According to Locke, this annuls the right to possess both the land and the food grown on it.

But rather than getting bogged down by a feeling of guilt, we should regard this tragic squandering of resources as a magnificent opportunity. We can reduce our environmental impact, while increasing the amount of food available, simply by eating less meat and not wasting food. A survey conducted in Australia in 2005 found that 60 percent of people felt guilty about buying and then wasting items such as food; only 14 percent of respondents said they were not much bothered or not bothered at all. But rather than feeling guilty, we should feel empowered by the sense of responsibility. It is a relief, in many ways, that we can enhance the lives of the world's hungry and reduce pressure on land by doing something so easy as eating more plant-based meals, buying only the food we are going to eat, and eating whatever we buy.

GROWING FOOD IN A COMMUNITY GARDEN

■ Karen Washington

Farmer and activist

Do you know where your food comes from? This is a question that everyone should be asking themselves and their family members. Did you also know that during the early 1900s, 40 percent of our population lived on farms? We had over 50 million farmers and over 500 million farms. Today, those numbers have drastically decreased to around 3.2 million farmers and 2 million farms. And yet, the actual farm size and production has increased due to industrialization and agribusiness. At the same time, our once plant-based diet has become increasingly more animal-based; as a result, our average caloric intake has gone from 2,000 calories to 3,800 calories per person. Is it any surprise that a food system that encourages such overabundance has resulted in a population of unhealthy and obese people?

I live in a low-income neighborhood in the Bronx section of New York City. I have seen firsthand the differences in the quality of food here. We are surrounded by fast-food chains and junk food. Politicians might call our neighborhood a food desert, but the real problem is hunger and poverty. We have plenty of food—what is lacking are nutritious food choices.

There are, however, people in cities across the country who are working to combat food inequality by growing their own. Here in New York, we have over 600 community gardens; in my borough alone there are close to 120. I started my garden, the Garden of Happiness, back in 1988. It was one of 15,000 vacant lots in New York at the time. Over the past few decades, community gardens of all shapes and sizes have become the lungs of the city. Each year people throughout New York's five boroughs grow tons of vegetables, herbs, and flowers. The majority of this bounty is grown in individual plots owned and maintained by a garden member.

When I first started the Garden of Happiness, I had no gardening experience. But I learned quickly by reading books and through word of mouth. I started by growing tomatoes, green peppers, and eggplant—and of course collard greens. As an African American, collards are part of my family's culture and tradition. Yet it was my first tomato that would change my attitude toward vegetables. The taste was incredible. It gave me the incentive to plant, grow, and eat all types of vegetables.

One advantage of growing food in a community garden is that you can grow your favorite vegetables. You plant a seed in the soil, water and nurture that seedling, and watch it thrive. Before you know it, it's time to collect your harvest. Often, the garden allows us an opportunity to plant vegetables not available in local supermarkets or bodegas. In fact, one of the best ways to try new and potentially unfamiliar kinds of vegetables and herbs is by trading with your neighbors. For instance, I have bartered for tastes of callaloo, tomatillos, cilantro, and Asian pears from my fellow gardeners. People often ask: What do we do with the excess produce? Most give it away or donate it to a local food pantry or soup kitchen. In my neighborhood's case, we run a farmer's market that generates income for the garden.

My community garden allows me to share good food and good culture with my neighbors. Controlling what you eat and growing your own food gives you power. So, if you ever have the opportunity to visit a community garden, stop by; you just might be surprised by what is growing inside.

HOW LANGUAGE, FOOD, AND IDENTITY INTERSECT

■ Samuel Boerboom

Editor of The Political Language of Food

What really is in a name? When it comes to the role food choices play in one's sense of self as a moral and political being, everything. The political language of food-based identities is greatly significant for those, like reducetarians and others, for whom food choices make up an embodied identity. Perhaps no choice we make is more embodied than that regarding what we eat. Eating habits are embodied commitments because we put our bodies in the choices we make and, just as important, in the persuasive language we use to describe those choices and ethical commitments. Language, food, and identity intersect in deeply meaningful ways. In this intersection we encounter how eating is fundamental to identity.

Sometimes described as microidentities, food-based identities are often anything but. To identify as reducetarian, for example, is not merely to describe one's diet but to offer one's body as proof of a coherent political identity that reflects one's commitment to the physical environment, human health and well-being, and the welfare of animals raised for human consumption. Language is inherently political and impacts significantly our food decisions. It can be difficult to make conscientious food choices—ones that reflect political conscience—because the food information environment on which we rely to make ethical choices about nourishing and sustainable food is often imprecise and confusing. Consumers receive inconsistent and contradictory information from regulatory agencies, food marketers, the scientific community, and the news media, which hinders informed food choices. One effect of this use of vague language is that food marketers and manufacturers profit from the halo effect of items labeled as "natural" or "wholesome."

Eaters who join up with one another under a common banner of a food-based identity do so in part to make sense of the confusion and to speak back to powerful food interests. In addition, much of the language used to describe a conscientious diet—vegetarian, vegan, conscientious carnivore—fails to capture the nuances or the political motivation for ethical eating. Ethical eating does not merely involve a commitment to one's health. It symbolizes, in ways perhaps no other political identity can, one's multifaceted ethical self. Identities like "liberal" or "libertarian," "humanist" or "believer" are abstract expressions of ethical and moral values. A diet-based identity, however, is a more concrete expression of one's values. After all, the food we consume is a foundational statement to who we are, what and whom we value. No more intimate and personally felt political expression can occur than one that is bodily enacted. We persuade not so much in what we say, but in what we do over and over again, with our bodies serving as proof. Knowingly or unknowingly, eaters express their political conscience each and every time they eat.

The language of one's food-based identity is essential to making known political commitments and for compelling others to identify with and share those commitments. It is likely that many eaters feel that food is crucial to their political identity, but they have until recently lacked the terminology to express it. While food language can unite eaters, it can just as easily divide. When well-meaning individuals attempt to distinguish their food identity from another, even when those two identities have overlapping values, they run the risk of losing political solidarity and the chance for achieving lasting outcomes. Structural change cannot happen when food organizations and social movements question the motives of those who do not fully agree with them. There are more food-based identities available for consideration than ever before. Indeed, food and our eating habits are increasingly central to understanding one's political self. Still, those food-based organizations and social movements that commit to welcoming others who share at least some of their values and goals are far more likely to endure and affect change than those who are parochial in outlook and exclusionary in promoting ethical eating habits.

Little is more fundamental than the deliberately political act of choosing how to feed ourselves and those we care about. Our bodies are sites of ongoing political decisions. The identities we choose and the language we use to express that choice tells a story that is deeply and necessarily political.

RECIPES

*So the pie isn't perfect? Cut it into wedges. Stay in control,
and never panic.*

—MARTHA STEWART

INTRODUCTION

■ Pat Crocker

"We eat to nourish our cells and we share meals with family and friends to nourish our lives. By taking an active interest in the way our food is grown and processed and in the way it is handled and prepared, served and enjoyed, we take back responsibility for not only our nourishment and health, but also that of the planet. And that alone is a powerful act." I penned those words in 2006 for my book *The Vegetarian Cook's Bible*, and they are especially appropriate as I set out to prepare a collection of kitchen basics and recipes for *The Reducetarian Solution*.

Reducetarian cooking is all about balance and harmony. It encompasses a relaxed approach to food and as such, it is spontaneous, simple, and playful and at the same time, it is deliciously healthy. Like the essays in this book, reducetarian recipes offer a serious solution that speaks to the issues surrounding our modern ways of feeding ourselves.

Why cook from scratch?

The reducetarian approach to cooking and eating compels you to rethink your food attitudes and replace them with two simple goals: to be aware of and begin to reduce the amount of meat you consume. I believe that to do this, you must be mindful and make conscious food decisions three, four, perhaps more times a day and physically act on them. Once you do that, the next steps are into the market and then the kitchen because it is only by preparing food yourself that you truly take control over what you eat. Home cooks prepare food differently from commercial, mostly mechanized systems because they use honest foods with no chemical preservatives or additives; and these kitchen heroes select and combine food with love and family needs in mind.

Cooking is one activity that keeps you present—it may be meditative or it may forge new interactions. Cooking is elemental to the human condition, and we all are the descendants of cooks. Preparing meals allows you to be of service to others, and it definitely is a way to show generosity, gratitude, and love toward yourself, your family, and friends. Experience has taught me that one's relationship with food begins with family and culture and those filters shape our thoughts, feelings, unconscious habits, and actions. Being mindful about food—with conscious, respectful selection, handling, combining, and cooking of it—is a humble way to break free of deep, mostly unconscious bonds that do not serve an enlightened way of being.

Food forms the nucleus of health, and ethical, sustainable, delicious, whole, and honest food is within almost everyone's grasp. It is my goal to inspire you to put the messages found in this book to a practical and very enjoyable way of fulfilling one of our most basic needs. It's not difficult. In fact, it is pretty simple: eat plants as close as possible to the way they grow. Choose from a wide range of colors. Fill up your plate with whole grains, vegetables, fruits, nuts, seeds, and herbs and use healthy oils sparingly (see "Stocking the Reducetarian Pantry"). Eliminate if you can, or simply reduce the amount of animal ingredients you add to recipes or to your plate.

What follows is a reducetarian primer, a "DIY guide" for people of every culinary skill level to get into the kitchen, sing, dance, and experience the sheer joy that comes with the sensory pleasure that is cooking. The recipes are straightforward and simple with flair and loads of flavor, and some reflect traditional ethnic combinations. They are designed so that you have lots of choice, and I hope you think of them as templates and use them as a platform from which you soar toward a new relationship with your spirit, your mind, body, and the green gem we call Earth.

THE REDUCETARIAN TOOLBOX

STOCKING THE REDUCETARIAN PANTRY

As you gradually sync with the movement away from unconscious dependency on meat, instead of feeling deprived, you may be awed by the wide and varied spectrum of plant ingredients and combinations that delight and satisfy. You may actually see that you were restricted by a meat-potatoes-vegetable regimen. Reducetarian thinking is expansive and inclusive, and it means you can be creative in how you choose to combine the following ingredients.

Fruit and vegetables	Plant foods contain a wide range of phytonutrients, both known and yet to be discovered. These vitamins, minerals, fiber, and other active components (including antioxidants and anti-inflammatories) are responsible for preventing disease and keeping us vibrant and healthy, but we get the best results from eating a wide range of colors and types of plants. Eat 6 to 10 servings per day in a rainbow of colors.
Beans, peas, and lentils	Fresh or dried beans (such as black, soy, fava, kidney, lima, garbanzo/chickpeas), peas (green, snow, snap, split, black- or brown-eyed), peanuts, and lentils (yellow, orange, green, black) provide plenty of plant protein, calcium, fiber, folate, iron, magnesium, phosphorus, potassium, riboflavin, thiamin, vitamin B_6, and zinc. See page 244 for directions on how to cook dried beans. Use legumes (beans, peas, peanuts, or lentils) to replace meat.
Nuts and seeds	Most nuts and seeds contain more than 60 percent heart-healthy monounsaturated fats, protein, fiber, B vitamins, vitamin E, and many other minerals and antioxidants. Add ½ to 1 cup to meatless dishes for the taste, texture, and nutrients.
Whole grains	Grains are the seeds of cereal grasses. Whole or "brown" grains, including spelt, Kamut, wheat, rye, amaranth, barley, quinoa (see page 249 for how to cook), and oats contain the nutrient-dense bran, endosperm, and germ of the kernel. Eat whole grains to add complex carbohydrates for energy along with fiber and nutrients.

Herbs and spices	A wealth of phytonutrients is concentrated in the leaves, flowers, stems, roots, and bark of the plants we call herbs and spices. Many, like garlic, chiles, and turmeric, offer powerful anticancer, antioxidant, and anti-inflammatory components. Protection from heart disease, Alzheimer's, and diabetes can be found in these flavorful ingredients. Add herbs and spices to every dish you cook and eat.
Polyunsaturated oils	Heart-healthy oils are the best. Find a good quality, extra-virgin olive, nut, or avocado oil, store it in the refrigerator and use it for low-heat cooking, salad dressings, and raw dishes. For all other cooking, use coconut oil because it is stable at higher temperatures and it is safe to store at room temperature. Heart-healthy fats and oils deserve a seat at the table—use them prudently.

EQUIPPING THE REDUCETARIAN KITCHEN

The vegan, vegetarian, or reducetarian kitchen is not very different from one that prepares meat. The point here is that mindfulness in equipping the kitchen means that you make decisions based on long-term usefulness: Get the best-quality tool you can afford. This means opting for stainless-steel cooking and prepping utensils and learning that fewer gadgets and less plastic means more in the reducetarian kitchen. Here are some of the items that will stand up well to everyday meal making. I've listed the essential items to get you started. As you expand your cooking curiosity and skills, you can add specific tools that you know you will use and enjoy.

Always look for quality, durability, and food-safe, environmentally friendly materials in kitchen equipment.

3 knives	I own 3 knives: a paring knife and a chef's (or French) knife, both with all-in-one stainless-steel handles. I sharpen them every week, and I tested them in my hand before purchasing them. A serrated bread knife completes the set.
Chopping boards	A couple of dishwasher-safe boards are handy for chopping vegetables. Keep a different colored one separate for preparing meat.

2 stainless-steel saucepans	One each: 2-quart and 3- or 4-quart will do almost everything. One lid is usually all you need at any given time.
10- or 12-inch skillet	I love my heavy cast-iron skillet, but it requires preseasoning and salt to clean it. For everyday cooking, I use a heavy-bottom stainless-steel sauté pan. Use low to medium heat and sauté (stir frequently) to prevent sticking.
Wok	A large (mine has a 15-inch inside diameter) carbon steel or stainless-steel wok is essential to the reducetarian kitchen. Try Asian markets or Chinatown before spending more at trendy kitchen shops.
9 by 13-inch baking dish	Plant-based combinations are often baked in a covered casserole dish. Choose from ceramic, enameled cast iron, or heavy-duty stainless steel.
1 or 2 rimmed baking sheets	Start with one sheet and add more if you are seriously into making cookies. Rimmed baking sheets are more versatile than rimless cookie sheets, but for baking cookies and pizza, rimless sheets make their removal easier.
12-well muffin tin	There are different sizes, so consider what size muffins or soufflés or other bite-size foods you want to bake. The 2-inch well size works for my needs.
Set of 3 mixing bowls	Ceramic, glass, or stainless-steel bowls are essential.
Measuring utensils	To accurately measure ingredients, you need a set of measuring spoons: (⅛-, ¼-, ½-, 1-teaspoon, and 1-tablespoon) and a set of dry measures: (¼-, ⅓-, ½-, and 1-cup). These should be high-quality stainless steel. In addition, a glass measuring cup is best for measuring liquids. It's good to have 1-, 2-, and 8-cup glass measures, but get the 2-cup liquid measure and add the other sizes as you need them.
Colander and/or strainer	To drain pasta, cooked beans, and other ingredients, you will need a stainless-steel colander. A strainer is lighter, with finer mesh, and it fits over bowls for straining smaller ingredients and saving the liquids.
2 long-handled spoons	One slotted and one regular stainless-steel spoon make mixing, transferring, and serving food easy.
2 wooden spoons	Long-handled bamboo or hardwood spoons keep your hand away from heat and are gentle on pans as you stir food on the stove.
2 spatulas	One large and one small spatula efficiently scrape food from bowls, pans, and cans.

Garlic press	Garlic is the king of herbs, and I use it every day. A good stainless-steel press with ergonomic handles makes fast work of mincing fresh cloves.
Flat, bowl graters	I prefer flat, stainless steel graters that fit over a bowl. Choose two (or three) sizes from small to large for grating cheese, vegetables, and salad ingredients.
Mandolin	Adjustable blade height slices firm fruit and vegetables evenly. Mine is small and sits over a medium bowl.
Blender or food processor	I use my food processor (for chopping, slicing, grating, and making pesto) more often than I do my blender, but having said that, a high-performance blender is useful for puréeing soup and sauce, and for smoothies.
Slow cooker	I use mine every week in the winter, and it keeps the oven off during summer. If you carve out a half hour in the morning before work to load it up, it sure is nice to come home to a hot, healthy dinner.
Egg beaters	I use a wire whisk for beating eggs and blending sauce ingredients and a hand-operated eggbeater to whip cream and beat a large quantity of eggs or egg whites. You will know when to add an electric beater and/or an immersion blender to your kitchen.

RECIPES

- V = vegan
- F = flex options are included
- GF = gluten free
- R = raw

TOOLBOX BASICS

- Garam Masala Spice Blend
- Green Herb Pesto
- Red Curry Paste

Garam Masala Spice Blend (V, GF)

I use this a few times a week because it is so good in casserole dishes and with grains, especially rice. The cinnamon makes it slightly sweet, and it isn't hot spicy. Purchase small quantities of fresh, whole spices whenever possible and grind them using a mortar and pestle or an electric spice or coffee grinder. This method dry-toasts the whole or crushed spices before grinding them. If making your own spice blend seems overwhelming, there are some very good blends available in stores and on the Internet.

Makes ½ cup

4 whole cloves
One 3-inch piece cinnamon, crushed
1 whole star anise, crushed
1 whole nutmeg, crushed
4 tablespoons coriander seeds
2 tablespoons cumin seeds
1 tablespoon black peppercorns
1 teaspoon cardamom seeds

1. Combine the cloves, cinnamon, star anise, nutmeg, coriander, cumin, peppercorns, and cardamom in a small dry skillet or spice wok. Toast the spices over medium heat, stirring frequently, until lightly browned and fragrant, 3 to 4 minutes. Watch carefully and remove from the heat just as the seeds begin to pop or the spices will smoke and burn. Set aside to cool.

2. Pound or grind the toasted spices to your desired consistency using a mortar and pestle or small electric grinder. Transfer to an airtight glass jar, label, and store in a cool, dark place. Use within 3 months.

Green Herb Pesto (GF, R)

Also known as salsa verde, to the French it is pistou. The word pesto *is derived from the Latin* pestare, *meaning "to pound or crush," which is also the source of the word* pestle, *the crushing tool used with a mortar. Use fresh basil leaves or any combination of green herbs, such as sage, thyme, tarragon, parsley, or bee balm. In the winter I use spinach, kale, and parsley and in the spring, I favor dandelion, sorrel, radish leaves, and chives or wild leeks. You can use the tops of garlic, known as scapes, or any other green that is in season to make this versatile sauce.*

Makes 2 cups

3 large garlic cloves
¼ cup sunflower seeds or nuts, such as pine, walnut, almond
¼ cup grated hard cheese such as Asiago, Parmesan, or Romano
2 cups fresh green leaves (see the recipe introduction)
¼ to ½ cup extra-virgin olive oil or avocado oil

1. Combine the garlic, seeds, and cheese in the bowl of a food processor. Process until finely chopped, about 1 minute. Add the leaves to the bowl. With the motor running, slowly add the oil through the opening in the lid. Keep adding oil until the sauce reaches your desired consistency. Transfer to an airtight glass jar, label, and store in the refrigerator for up to 2 weeks.

Red Curry Paste (V, GF, R)

A good curry blend is one that you develop over time by experimenting. Not hot enough? Add more cayenne or chipotle. Too spicy? Increase the paprika and coriander . . . and so it goes until you have a blend tailored to suit your cooking style. You can purchase curry powder, but try this rich and complex blend of fresh chiles and spices for authentic Asian flavors. Pastes are easy to use in cooking because they blend into liquids (broth and coconut milk) for instant results. Use 1 or 2 tablespoons of this paste as a substitute whenever curry powder or Garam Masala Spice Blend (page 231) is called for.

Makes 1 scant cup

4 garlic cloves, minced
2 red chile peppers, finely chopped
1 stalk fresh lemongrass, white part only, minced
¼ medium red onion, chopped
3 tablespoons coconut milk, or as needed
2 tablespoons tomato paste or chili sauce
2 tablespoons tamari or soy sauce
2 tablespoons freshly squeezed lime juice
1 tablespoon grated fresh ginger
1 tablespoon paprika
1 teaspoon ground cumin
1 teaspoon granulated sugar
½ teaspoon ground coriander
¼ teaspoon ground cinnamon
¼ teaspoon ground white pepper

1. Combine all of the ingredients in the bowl of a food processor or blender container. Process or blend on high until well blended, about 1 minute. Add more coconut milk if the paste is too thick. Transfer to a jar, cap, and store in the refrigerator for up to 1 week.

LITE BITES (BREAKFAST, LUNCH, LATE-NIGHT DISHES)

- Buffalo Cauliflower
- Cheesy Apple Pancakes
- Grilled Portobello Stack
- Mushrooms on Toast
- Nutty Bean Pitas
- Eat the Rainbow Pizza
- Tofu Scramble

Buffalo Cauliflower (V-Option, GF)

Here's a tasty way to replace chicken wings. Heat up the action off the field during the Super Bowl with these cheesy-spicy bites. You can use ½ cup sunflower seeds in place of the cheese for a vegan option.

Makes 4 light servings

1 cauliflower, cut into 1-inch florets
1½ teaspoons sea salt, divided
2 tablespoons extra-virgin coconut oil or olive oil
1 onion, chopped
1 jalapeño pepper, finely chopped
2 garlic cloves, finely chopped
1 tablespoon Garam Masala Spice Blend (page 231) or Red Curry
    Paste (page 233)
½ cup large-flake rolled oats
1 cup grated Parmesan cheese, optional

1. Preheat the oven to 400°F. Lightly oil an 11 by 17-inch roasting pan.

2. Place the cauliflower in a large saucepan and cover with water. Add 1 teaspoon of the salt and bring to a boil over medium-high heat. Reduce heat to medium and boil just until stems are tender-crisp, about 5 minutes. Drain, rinse with cool water, and drain again. Set aside.

3. Meanwhile, heat the oil in a skillet over medium-high heat. Add the onion and sauté until soft and fragrant, about 6 minutes. Add the pepper, garlic, and spice blend. Cook, stirring frequently, 2 minutes. Turn the heat off and add the oats and remaining ½ teaspoon of salt. Toss to mix well.

4. Toss the cauliflower and onion mixture in the prepared pan until combined. Roast about 10 minutes or until the edges start to darken. Sprinkle with cheese if using and return to the oven for 2 minutes or until the cheese has melted.

Cheesy Apple Pancakes

These puffy griddlecakes are easy and fast and satisfyingly good. Serve piping hot with fresh fruit or frozen yogurt for dessert, or add a dollop of the ricotta cheese with slices of banana and drizzle with maple syrup for a hearty breakfast. For lunch or dinner, smear them with Green Herb Pesto (page 232) or Bean Spread (page 244) and top with thinly sliced carrot, cucumber, cabbage, and red onion and serve with a salad. For a totally leftover lunch, place a spoonful of any leftover main dish in the center, roll up, and eat like a burrito.

Makes 6 to 8 pancakes

½ cup drained ricotta or cottage cheese
1 apple, shredded
2 large eggs, lightly beaten
2 tablespoons maple syrup or honey
1 teaspoon vanilla extract
½ cup whole wheat or all-purpose flour
1 teaspoon baking soda
1 teaspoon ground cinnamon
½ teaspoon sea salt
1 to 2 tablespoons extra-virgin olive oil or coconut oil

1. Preheat the oven to 300°F.

2. Combine the cheese, apple, eggs, maple syrup, and vanilla in a medium bowl. Whisk with a fork until well mixed.

3. Combine the flour, baking soda, cinnamon, and salt in a large bowl. Pour the cheese mixture into the flour mixture and whisk with a fork just until incorporated. Do not over mix.

4. Lightly oil a griddle or large skillet and heat over medium-high heat. Scoop the batter using a ¼-cup measure (for small cakes) or ½-cup measure (for medium cakes) and scrape onto the hot griddle, spreading each pancake to about ½-inch thickness. Cook until the bottom is golden and large bubbles form on the uncooked side, about 2 minutes. Flip and cook the remaining side until golden, about 2 minutes.

5. Remove cooked pancakes to a plate, cover with foil, and keep warm in preheated oven. Repeat step 4 using remaining batter.

Grilled Portobello Stack (V-Option, F)

It's like a decadent, oozing burger, full of texture and flavor, and yet it is deliciously, perfectly in line with reducetarian principles. You can use sliced tomato or dill pickle in place of the avocado. Add a slice or two of bacon for a flex option, but really? I guarantee you won't miss the meat.

Makes 4 stacks

4 large Portobello mushrooms, cleaned and stemmed
1 small eggplant, peeled and cut into ½-inch slices crosswise
¼ cup extra-virgin olive or avocado oil
4 slices mozzarella or fontina cheese, optional
4 slices whole grain bread
½ cup Walnut-Olive Pesto (recipe follows) or Green Herb Pesto
    (page 232)
½ avocado, cut into slices
Sea salt and freshly ground black pepper to taste
4 to 8 slices bacon, cooked, optional

1. Preheat the oven to 400°F. Lightly grease a rimmed baking sheet.

2. Arrange the mushrooms, gill side down, on the prepared baking sheet. Add the eggplant slices in one layer and drizzle 3 tablespoons of the oil over all. Roast 15 minutes. Using a fork or tongs, flip the vegetables over and drizzle the remaining 1 tablespoon oil over all. Roast 15 minutes or until soft. Remove the eggplant to a plate and set aside. Top the 4 mushrooms (now gill side up) with a slice of cheese and return to the oven for 2 minutes or until cheese has melted.

3. Toast the bread and place on a work surface. Divide the walnut pesto evenly among the slices and spread to an even layer. Place a slice of eggplant over the pesto and layer on 1 or 2 slices of bacon if using and then a mushroom with melted cheese. Top each stack with a slice of avocado. Season with salt and pepper.

Walnut-Olive Pesto (V, F-Option, GF, R)

Makes ½ cup

½ cup walnut halves or pieces
¼ cup pitted black olives
1 tablespoon fresh thyme leaves
3 tablespoons extra-virgin olive oil or avocado oil, or to taste
Sea salt to taste

1. Combine the walnuts, olives, and thyme in the bowl of a food processor or blender container. Pulse until coarsely chopped, about 10 seconds. With the motor running, add the oil through the opening in the lid and process just until combined. Use more or less oil to make the pesto spreadable. Scrape into a small bowl and set aside. You can make this up to 3 days ahead and store, covered in the refrigerator. Bring to room temperature before using.

Mushrooms on Toast (V, GF-Option)

This is my go-to recipe for lunch or a light dinner when time and creative effort are at a low. It will be on the table in less than 20 minutes, and everyone in my house loves it. Teamed with a green salad or the Vegetable Slaw on page 253, it makes a well-rounded meal. You can add, and heat through, 1 cup of cooked legumes at the end of step 4.

Makes 4 servings

2 tablespoons coconut oil

1 onion, chopped

¼ red cabbage, chopped

½ red bell pepper, chopped

1 cayenne pepper, finely chopped, optional

5 cups chopped mushrooms

2 garlic cloves

1 tablespoon finely chopped fresh rosemary

½ teaspoon sea salt

4 slices whole grain, wheat, or gluten-free bread

1. Heat the oil in a large skillet over medium-high heat. Add the onion and sauté until soft, 5 minutes. Add the cabbage, bell pepper, and cayenne pepper if using. Cook, stirring frequently, about 3 minutes.

2. Stir in the mushrooms, garlic, rosemary, and salt and cook, stirring frequently until the mushrooms are tender, about 5 minutes, or until vegetables are soft.

3. Meanwhile, toast the bread and place it on plates. Divide the mushroom mixture evenly into 4 portions and spoon over the toast.

Nutty Bean Pitas (GF-Option)

Greek flavors combine to make these tasty pitas.

Makes 4 servings

1½ cups cooked fava or lima beans

1 garlic clove, finely chopped

1 tablespoon chopped fresh oregano or Green Herb Pesto (page 232)

¼ cup extra-virgin olive oil or avocado oil

½ cup chopped almonds or pistachio nuts

½ cup crumbled feta or soft goat cheese

Sea salt and freshly ground black pepper to taste

4 large whole grain, wheat, or gluten-free pitas (8 or 10 inches)

½ cucumber, coarsely shredded

¼ red onion, thinly sliced

1 tomato, seeded and chopped

Juice of 1 lemon

1. Preheat the oven to 375°F.

2. Combine beans, garlic, oregano, and 3 tablespoons of the oil in a large bowl. Mash using a potato masher or fork until the mixture is the consistency of a rough paste. Stir in the nuts and cheese and season with salt and pepper.

3. Cut the pitas in half and open to form pockets. Divide the bean mixture among the 8 pita halves and spread in an even layer over one side. Divide the cucumber, onion, and tomato evenly among the pita halves, stuffing the vegetables into each pocket. Drizzle each with the remaining 1 tablespoon oil and the lemon juice.

4. Arrange the pita halves on a baking sheet and cover with foil. Bake in preheated oven until warmed through, about 10 minutes.

Eat the Rainbow Pizza (V-Option, F-Option)

If you're thinking that pizza is fast food, here's a way to slow it down, entertain family and friends, and enjoy a plant-based treat. Kids love this and it keeps them busy for quite a while. The only recipe you need is for the pizza dough and if you purchase the dough, then all you really need to do is invent the sauce and toppings and start rolling. If you own a bread machine, follow the manufacturer's recipe for making pizza dough.

Handmade Pizza Dough

> **Makes 1 large (12-slice) or 2 medium (6-slice) or 3 small (4-slice) pizzas**
>
> 1 cup warm water (120°F)
> 1 package (2¼ teaspoons) active dry yeast
> 3 tablespoons extra-virgin olive oil, plus more for brushing
>   the dough
> 3 cups bread or all-purpose flour, plus more for kneading
> 2 teaspoons sugar
> 1 teaspoon sea salt
> Cornmeal for dusting
> Sauce, cheese, and toppings (see chart on page 241)

1. Bring all the ingredients and utensils except the water to room temperature. Place the water in a measuring cup or small bowl. Add sugar and stir until dissolved. Sprinkle the yeast over top and set aside until the yeast is dissolved and foamy, about 5 minutes. Add the oil and stir well.

2. Combine flour and salt in a large bowl. Using a wooden spoon, gradually stir in the water-yeast mixture. When all of the liquid has been added, turn out the dough onto a lightly floured surface.

3. Lightly dust your hands with flour and, using your hands, mix and knead the dough, adding flour, 1 tablespoon at a time as needed, until the dough is smooth and elastic, about 8 minutes.

4. Wash and dry the mixing bowl and lightly oil it. Place the dough in the bowl and flip it over so the top is lightly oiled. Cover with a clean cloth or plastic wrap and set aside in a warm place to rise until it has doubled in size, about 1 hour.

5. Preheat the oven to 450°F. Punch the dough down, form into one round ball. Cut the dough into 2 equal balls, wrap each in plastic, and set them aside to rest for 10 minutes.

6. Sprinkle 1 tablespoon of cornmeal over the work surface. Roll out one ball of dough, thin or thick (¼ to ½ inch thick). Transfer the dough to a baking sheet and let it rest for 10 minutes. Press from the center toward the edges to form a slightly raised rim.

7. Brush the top of the pizza dough with 1 teaspoon of olive oil. Spoon 2 to 3 tablespoons sauce over and sprinkle about ¼ cup cheese over. Top with a rainbow of vegetables and other ingredients. Bake until the crust is golden brown and the cheese is bubbly, 10 to 15 minutes.

8. Repeat steps 6 and 7 if using the second ball of dough. If not using the second ball of dough, wrap tightly and refrigerate for up to 2 days or freeze for up to 3 months.

SAUCE SUGGESTIONS 3 tablespoons	CHEESE SUGGESTIONS 3 to 4 tablespoons	TOPPING SUGGESTIONS ⅓ cup	OTHER INGREDIENTS 2 tablespoons
Baba Ghanoush (page 243)	Shredded mozzarella	GREEN VEGGIES: broccoli, fresh greens (dandelion, shredded kale, arugula), shaved Brussels sprouts, chopped asparagus, pea sprouts, fresh peas	Chopped nuts
Green Herb Pesto (page 232)	Sliced fresh buffalo mozzarella		Chopped seeds
barbecue sauce	Crumbled feta		Crumbled tempeh
Béchamel sauce	Crumbled blue		CHOPPED FRESH HERBS: rosemary, basil, oregano, thyme
Fruit Salsa (page 264)	Shredded cheddar	RED VEGGIES: sliced tomatoes, shredded carrot, chopped red pepper, shredded red cabbage, diced hot peppers	
Garlic oil (1 garlic clove, minced, and 3 tablespoons extra-virgin olive oil)	Shredded fontina or Havarti		Marinated tofu cubes
	Shredded Romano or Parmesan		Olives
Guacamole (page 245)		WHITE VEGGIES: sliced onion, sliced fennel, sliced radishes, sliced mushrooms, shredded turnip, grilled sliced eggplant, sliced leeks, sliced radishes	
Bean Spread (page 244)			
Mushroom sauce			
Tomato Sauce (page 266)		FRUIT: chopped figs, plums, grapes, pineapple, strawberries,	
Walnut-Olive Pesto (page 237)		MEAT: Smoked or cooked chicken pieces, sliced prosciutto, crumbled cooked bacon, chopped sausage, Parma Ham Crisps (page 246)	

Tofu Scramble (V, GF)

Freezing tofu gives it an extra-chewy texture and if you have frozen tofu, remove it from the freezer, place in a bowl, and defrost in the refrigerator overnight. Once thawed, set the tofu aside for an hour in a colander in the sink to drain before proceeding with the recipe. It's worth the extra time for the toothiness it imparts to this dish.

Makes 4 servings

1 block (14-ounce) extra-firm tofu (see recipe introduction)

2 tablespoons extra-virgin olive oil or coconut oil

1 onion, chopped

1 red bell pepper, chopped

1 small zucchini, chopped, or 2 cups chopped kale

1 tablespoon Garam Masala Spice Blend (page 231) or Red Curry
      Paste (page 233)

2 cups cooked black beans, rinsed and drained

Sea salt and freshly ground black pepper to taste

4 wheat or corn tortillas, warmed

1 cup tomato salsa or Guacamole (page 245), optional

1. Place the tofu on a paper towel–lined plate and cover with a clean kitchen towel. Place something heavy on top (like a large can of vegetables or a cast iron skillet) and set aside to drain.

2. Heat the oil in a medium skillet over medium-high heat. Add the onion and sauté until soft, about 5 minutes. Stir in the bell pepper and zucchini and cook, stirring frequently, until vegetables are tender-crisp, about 5 minutes.

3. Using a fork, shred the tofu into small pieces. Add the tofu, spice blend, and beans to the onions. Cook, stirring frequently, until the beans and tofu are heated through, 1 to 2 minutes. Season with salt and pepper and serve with warmed tortillas and salsa if using.

SNACKS (IN-HAND FOOD, DIPS, SPREADS)

- Baba Ghanoush
- Bean Spread (Hummus)
- Guacamole
- Lettuce Wraps + Parma Ham
- Sweet Potato Fritters

Baba Ghanoush (GF)

If you have a blender or food processor, you can use it to purée the dip, but a potato masher works just fine. Roasting the garlic caramelizes the sugars and adds to the smoky taste of the charred eggplant. Tahini sauce is ground sesame seeds with their oil. Mix the oil into the paste before measuring for recipes.

Makes 2 cups

2 medium eggplants
1 whole head garlic
3 tablespoons extra-virgin olive oil or coconut oil
Juice and grated rind of 1 lemon
1 cup Greek yogurt or drained plain yogurt
⅓ cup tahini sauce
Sea salt and freshly ground black pepper to taste
Toasted pita triangles or bagel chips
Assorted cut-up raw vegetables

1. Set the top oven rack to the highest position. Preheat the oven to broil (500°F).

2. Pierce the eggplants all over with a fork and place on a rimmed baking sheet. Slice ¼ inch off the top of the head of garlic and rub the loose skin away from the outside of the head. Place on the baking sheet, cut side up, and drizzle the top with 1 tablespoon of the oil.

3. Broil, turning the eggplants once or twice, until the eggplants collapse and the flesh of the eggplants and garlic are very soft. Set aside to cool, about 40 minutes. Pour any seeping liquids into a large bowl.

4. When cool, slice the eggplants in half lengthwise and scrape the pulp into the bowl, discarding the skins. Separate the cloves of garlic and squeeze the flesh of each into the bowl. Mash using a potato masher. Add the remaining 2 tablespoons of oil, the lemon rind, lemon juice, yogurt, and tahini sauce. Mix well. Season with salt and pepper. Serve with pita triangles and vegetables.

Bean Spread (Hummus) (V, GF)

I give the method for cooking dried beans here, and once you make them, you'll see how easy it is to have cooked beans on hand to enrich the plant protein in all sorts of dishes. If you are using the beans for a spread or dip, cook them until soft, otherwise for salads and soups or other cooked dishes, cook them just until tender and add to the dish in the last minutes of cooking.

You may choose to stock cooked canned beans for convenience, but be sure that there is no BPA (a chemical used in plastic food containers and tin linings). If it doesn't have the "BPA-free" claim on the label, the food may contain levels of up to 200 times government guidelines for safe exposure.

How to Cook Dried Beans from Scratch

Makes about 3 cups cooked beans

1 cup raw, dried beans (chickpeas, red or black kidney beans, or
   other variety, sorted and washed)
6 cups water

1. Put the beans and water in a large saucepan or stockpot and bring to a boil over high heat. Cover, reduce the heat, and simmer 2 minutes. Turn the heat off, leave the pot on the burner, and let sit for 1 hour.

2. Drain, rinse, and return the beans to the saucepan. Fill the pan with cool water until it rises 2 inches over the top of the beans. Bring to a boil over high heat. Reduce the heat and simmer uncovered until tender, 60 to 90 minutes. Drain, rinse, and pat dry. Transfer the beans to a lidded container or zip-top bag and store in the refrigerator for up to 5 days or freeze for up to 3 months.

■ *Bean Spread*
As always, you are in control: add more liquids for a dip or less liquids to achieve a thicker spread.

Makes 3 cups

2 cups cooked beans
1 cup finely chopped walnuts
2 garlic cloves, minced
½ cup tahini sauce
Juice and grated rind of 1 lemon
1 to 2 tablespoons extra-virgin olive oil or coconut oil
1 teaspoon tamari or soy sauce
Sea salt and freshly ground black pepper to taste

1. Mash the beans in a large bowl. Add the walnuts, garlic, tahini sauce, lemon juice, lemon rind, oil, and tamari. Taste and add salt and pepper as required.

Guacamole (V, GF, R)

A basic recipe for guacamole is given here, but because there are so many ingredients that can be added, I've listed some of them after the recipe. This recipe requires no electricity and cleanup is easy.

Makes 2 cups

2 ripe avocados
Juice and grated rind of 1 lemon
3 garlic cloves, chopped fine
½ teaspoon sea salt
¼ teaspoon powdered chipotle chile peppers

1. Starting at the top end slit an avocado lengthwise in half and twist to separate the halves. Using a spoon remove and discard the pit. Hold one half of an avocado in the palm of your hand, cut end up, and slip the spoon between the flesh and the skin to remove the flesh, discarding the skin. Roughly chop and place in a medium bowl. Drizzle the lemon juice over. Remove the skin from the second half and add chopped avocado flesh to the bowl and toss to coat with lemon juice. Repeat with the second avocado.

2. Mash the avocados using a potato masher. Add the lemon rind, garlic, salt, and chipotle powder. Stir well and add other suggested ingredients if desired.

Other Ingredients
　1 chopped hard-cooked egg
　½ small tomato seeded and chopped
　¼ cup chopped fresh chives
　¼ cup shredded and drained onion or cucumber
　¼ cup shredded carrot, rutabaga, celeriac, or beet
　¼ cup finely chopped green or red bell pepper
　¼ cup chopped olives
　⅓ cup mayonnaise`
　⅓ cup Greek yogurt or drained plain yogurt
　⅓ cup sour cream
　3 tablespoons finely chopped fresh cilantro, parsley, or oregano

Lettuce Wraps (V, GF) + Parma Ham Crisps (F)

Make these exceptional wraps seasonal by using spring asparagus, fresh green peas in summer, chopped kale in fall, and a hearty green such as chopped cabbage or thinly sliced Brussels sprouts in winter. Serve the Parma Ham Crisps inside the wrap or on the side for a flex option.

■ *Parma Ham Crisps*

Makes ¼ pound

　¼ pound sliced Parma ham

1. Preheat the oven to 450°F. Line a rimmed baking sheet with parchment paper.

2. Place the ham slices in one layer on the prepared baking sheet. Bake until crisp, 3 to 5 minutes. Using tongs, transfer the slices to a towel-lined plate and set aside.

■ *Wraps*

   1 head Boston, Bibb, or butter lettuce
   4 ounces rice cellophane noodles
   2 tablespoons extra-virgin olive oil or coconut oil
   1 large onion, chopped
   1 red bell pepper, chopped
   2 garlic cloves, finely chopped
   1 tablespoon tamari or soy sauce
   1 tablespoon rice wine vinegar
   1 can (6 ounces) water chestnuts, drained and chopped
   1 cup chopped cooked greens (see recipe introduction)
   ¼ cup coarsely chopped salted peanuts or pistachio nuts

1. Core the lettuce and rinse under cool water. Drain and pat dry. Remove 8 leaves and place on a clean kitchen towel in the crisper section of the refrigerator until ready to use.

2. Place the noodles in a medium bowl and add boiling water to cover. Set aside until soft, 12 to 15 minutes. Drain and set aside.

3. Heat the oil in a medium skillet over medium-high heat. Add the onion and sauté about 5 minutes. Add the bell pepper and garlic and cook, stirring frequently, until the vegetables are soft, about 5 minutes. Add the tamari, vinegar, water chestnuts, and greens. Cook, stirring frequently, to heat through, about 1 minute. Use tongs to hold the noodles over the skillet and cut roughly into 2-inch lengths, letting the pieces fall into the pan. Remove the skillet from the heat, add the nuts, and toss to combine. Transfer to a serving bowl.

4. Arrange the lettuce leaves into 2 stacks on one side of a large serving platter. Place the ham on the other side and transfer the noodle mixture to the center. Diners can then fill and wrap their own lettuce cups.

Sweet Potato Fritters (V-Option, GF)

The eggs act as a binding agent in this recipe. To replace them with a plant alternative, mix 3 tablespoons chia seeds with ½ cup warm water. Set aside until the mixture is thick and egg-like in texture, 3 to 5 minutes.

Makes 4 to 6 servings

1 cup shredded sweet potato
1 cup shredded white potato
½ cup shredded carrot or parsnip
½ onion, finely chopped
1 cup shredded cheddar cheese, optional
½ cup chickpea flour or all-purpose flour
¼ teaspoon ground nutmeg
Sea salt and freshly ground black pepper to taste
2 eggs, beaten (see recipe introduction)
4 tablespoons extra-virgin olive oil or coconut oil

1. Place the shredded sweet and white potato in a colander in the sink and set aside to drain for 10 to 20 minutes.

2. Combine the drained potatoes, carrot, onion, cheese if using, flour, nutmeg, salt, and pepper in a large bowl. Toss to combine well. Stir in the eggs.

3. Preheat the oven to 325°F.

4. Heat 2 tablespoons of the oil in a large skillet over medium-high heat. Working in batches, drop the potato mixture by the ¼ cup into the hot pan. Reduce the heat to medium and cook until golden on the underside, 5 to 7 minutes. Flip the fritters over and cook 2 to 3 minutes. Transfer the fritters to an ovenproof plate and keep warm in the oven. Repeat with the remaining potato mixture and oil.

DINNER IN A BOWL
- Berry-Bean and Quinoa Salad
- Hot Potato Salad
- Roasted Beet Soup

- Slow Cooked Moroccan Carrot Soup
- Vegetable Slaw

Berry-Bean and Quinoa Salad (V, GF)

With its pleasant nutty taste and high protein, fiber, and minerals, quinoa is the perfect reducetarian grain. Cook more than you need for this recipe—you can double the recipe—so that you can refrigerate or freeze the remaining cooked grain to add to almost every recipe in this primer: wraps, salads, soup, stew, and even pizza.

How to Cook Quinoa

Makes 2 cups

1 cup red, black, or golden quinoa
2 teaspoons extra-virgin olive oil
2 cups water or vegetable broth
½ teaspoon sea salt

1. Place the quinoa in a fine mesh strainer and rinse under cool running water for about 2 minutes, rubbing and swishing the quinoa with your hand. Drain.

2. Heat the oil in a medium saucepan over medium-high heat. Add the quinoa and cook, stirring constantly, 1 minute.

3. Add the water and salt and bring to a boil. Reduce the heat to low, cover, and cook 15 minutes. Remove from the heat and let stand, covered, 5 minutes.

Dressing

Makes about 3/4 cup

4 tablespoons extra-virgin olive oil or avocado oil
Juice and grated rind of 1 lemon
2 teaspoons toasted sesame oil
1 tablespoon tamari or soy sauce

Salad

Makes 4 to 6 servings

2 cups cooked quinoa

2 cups cooked beans (see How to Cook Dried Beans from Scratch
     on page 244)

2 cups torn fresh greens (spinach, kale, Swiss chard, arugula, or
     dandelion

½ cup dried blueberries or cherries, chopped

½ red onion, thinly sliced

½ red bell pepper, thinly sliced

¼ cup pomegranate seeds

1. Make the dressing: Place the olive oil, lemon juice, lemon rind, sesame oil, and tamari in a jar with a tight-fitting lid. Cap the jar and shake well to mix.

2. Make the salad: Place the quinoa, beans, greens, blueberries, onion, bell pepper, and pomegranate seeds in a large bowl. Toss to mix. To serve immediately, shake the dressing, drizzle over the salad, and toss to mix well.

3. To serve later, keep the salad and dressing separate, cover each, and store in the refrigerator for up to 1 day. When ready to serve, bring both to room temperature, then shake the dressing, drizzle over the salad, and toss to mix well.

Hot Potato Salad (V, GF, F-Option)

Sometimes I cook beans or rice or potatoes in the morning before work. You can prepare many staples on the weekend and keep, tightly covered, in the refrigerator for weekday meals. Adding beans, nuts, seeds, and other cooked vegetables—such as broccoli, cauliflower, carrots, peas, and Brussels sprouts—extend this side dish into a meal.

Makes 4 servings

4 medium potatoes

1 or 2 slices thick-sliced bacon per serving, flex option

3 tablespoons extra-virgin olive oil or coconut oil

1 large onion, chopped

2 garlic cloves, finely chopped

1 tablespoon Garam Masala Spice Blend (page 231)

1 tablespoon chopped fresh rosemary

2 tablespoons freshly squeezed lemon juice

¼ cup crumbled feta cheese or vegan substitute

Sea salt and freshly ground black pepper to taste

¼ cup sunflower seeds

1. Cook the potatoes in a large pot of boiling water over high heat until tender, about 25 minutes. Drain, rinse with cold water, and set aside to cool. When cool enough to handle, peel the potatoes, cover loosely, and set aside.

1A. The Flex Option: Preheat the oven to 450°F. Place the bacon on a rimmed baking sheet and bake 4 minutes. Flip the bacon and bake until browned and crisp, about 3 minutes. Transfer to a paper towel–lined plate and set aside to cool.

2. Heat the oil in a skillet over medium-high heat. Add the onion and sauté 5 minutes. Add the garlic and spice blend and cook, stirring frequently, until the garlic is fragrant but not colored, about 3 minutes. Add the lemon juice and stir, scraping up the browned onion bits.

3. Cut the potatoes into chunks and add to the skillet. Cook, stirring, until heated through, 1 to 3 minutes.

4. Stir in the cheese, turn the heat off, and leave the skillet on the burner, stirring occasionally, until the cheese has melted slightly but not completely, 2 to 3 minutes. Season with salt and pepper. Divide the potatoes evenly among 4 plates and garnish each with 1 tablespoon of sunflower seeds.

4A. The Flex Option: Crumble the bacon and sprinkle over the flex servings.

Roasted Beet Soup (V, GF)

Roasting all vegetables, but especially beets, is one of the tastiest ways to cook them. To prepare beets for cooking, scrub well using a vegetable brush. Trim away the top and bottom and, using a vegetable peeler, remove the top one third of the rough skin.

Makes 4 to 6 servings

4 medium beets, prepared (see recipe introduction) and quartered

2 carrots, cut into 1-inch chunks

1 onion, quartered

1 parsnip, cut into 1-inch chunks

6 unpeeled garlic cloves

4 tablespoons extra-virgin olive oil or coconut oil

Sea salt and freshly ground pepper to taste

¼ cup chopped fresh dill

1 can (28 ounces) chopped tomatoes and juices

2 cups vegetable broth

1 cup shredded cabbage

¾ cup sour cream, optional

1. Preheat the oven to 400°F. Toss the beets, carrots, onion, parsnip, garlic, and oil in a large bowl until combined. Spread the vegetables in one layer on one or two rimmed baking sheets. Roast until tender, about 40 minutes. Season with salt, pepper, and dill.

2. Meanwhile, place the tomatoes, their juices, and the broth in a large saucepan and bring to a boil over medium-high heat. Add the cabbage, reduce the heat to medium-low, and simmer, stirring occasionally, until the cabbage is soft, about 12 minutes. Squeeze the roasted garlic into the tomato mixture, discarding the skins. Stir in the roasted vegetables.

3. Remove the pan from the heat. Using an immersion blender, purée the vegetables until smooth, or, working in batches, transfer the soup to a blender container or food processor bowl and process until smooth. Return the soup to the pan and heat through. Garnish each serving with 2 tablespoons of sour cream if desired.

Slow Cooked Moroccan Carrot Soup (V, GF)

Pulses (aka dried peas or lentils) are high in plant protein, so cook and add them to vegan and vegetarian dishes liberally. Lentils are easy to cook because they don't require presoaking as do dried beans. Like beans, there are many different varieties from tiny, black "pearl" lentils, to larger brown, red, yellow, and green types. I keep a jar of lentils on hand in my pantry and add a cup to most soup and stew recipes.

Makes 4 to 6 servings

6 carrots, sliced
1 cup red or yellow lentils, sorted and washed
1 onion, chopped
2 garlic cloves, finely chopped
1 tablespoon grated fresh ginger
1 tablespoon Garam Masala Spice Blend (page 231)
4 cups vegetable broth
2 cans (15 ounces) coconut milk
Sea salt and freshly ground black pepper to taste

1. Place the carrots, lentils, onion, garlic, ginger, and spice blend in the crock of a slow cooker. Stir in the broth and coconut milk.

2. Cover and cook on low until the vegetables are tender, 6 to 8 hours.

3. Serve chunky or, working in batches, transfer the soup to a blender container or food processor bowl and process until smooth. Return the soup to a pan and heat through. Season with salt and pepper.

Vegetable Slaw (V, GF, R)

The dressing is important here, not only because it adds incredible flavor but also because it is made from scratch. Use it as a mayonnaise substitute in sandwiches and other dishes. Because it contains natural preservative ingredients (vinegar, coconut oil, and garlic), it keeps for several weeks in a covered jar in the refrigerator. Make double the amount and bring to room temperature before using.

On the weekend or at the beginning of the week, I double the slaw ingredi-
ents and combine them in a large zip-top bag. By squeezing out all of the
air before sealing the bag, the prepared vegetables stay bright and crisp in
the refrigerator for 5 days. I can add vegetables by the cup to soup, stew, or
other cooked dishes and drastically reduce prep time or I can have a salad
ready in the time it takes to toss the dressing with the vegetables.

Makes 4 to 6 servings

Dressing

¼ cup creamy cashew or peanut butter

3 tablespoons rice wine vinegar

2 tablespoons extra-virgin olive oil

2 tablespoons tamari or soy sauce

2 tablespoons coconut nectar or liquid honey

1 garlic clove, minced

1 tablespoon shredded fresh ginger

Slaw

2 cups sliced green cabbage

2 cups sliced red cabbage

2 apples, shredded

1 red or green bell pepper, thinly sliced

¼ red onion, thinly sliced

1. Make the dressing: Combine the nut butter, vinegar, oil, tamari, coconut nectar, garlic, and ginger in a medium bowl and whisk with a fork until well mixed.

2. Make the slaw: Place the green and red cabbage, apples, bell pepper, and onion in a large bowl, tossing to combine. To serve immediately, add the dressing and toss to mix well.

3. To serve later, keep slaw and dressing separate (see recipe introduction), cover each, and store in the refrigerator for up to 5 days. When ready to serve, bring both to room temperature, then whisk the dressing, drizzle dressing over the slaw, and toss to mix well. If serving the slaw within 24 hours, toss the slaw and dressing together, cover, and refrigerate. Bring to room temperature before serving.

GRAINS

- Corn Bread
- Pasta Primavera or Pasta Bolognese
- Soba Noodles with Pistachio Leeks + Scallops
- Vegetable Risotto + Ham
- Whole Grain–Greens Stir-Fry

Corn Bread (GF-Option, F-Option, V-Option)

Enjoy this classic, quick-rise bread in about 40 minutes from start to table. It can be served at any meal—from morning to night—and many variations make it a flexible staple. For example, pour the batter into a lightly oiled 12-cup muffin pan for individual servings, or add 2 cups corn kernels, 1 cup grated sharp cheddar cheese, ½ cup cooked crumbled Parma ham or bacon, and 1 finely chopped jalapeño pepper for a Southwestern twist; or stir in ½ cup hot salsa, leftover Tofu Scramble (page 241), or ¼ cup Guacamole (page 245).

Makes one 8-inch loaf

1 cup yellow cornmeal
1 cup all-purpose flour or gluten-free flour blend
1 tablespoon baking powder
½ teaspoon baking soda
¼ teaspoon sea salt
1 cup buttermilk or almond milk
1 egg or egg alternative
¼ cup liquid honey or coconut nectar
3 tablespoons extra-virgin coconut oil or butter, melted

1. Preheat the oven to 425°F. Lightly oil an 8 by 8-inch baking pan.

2. Place the cornmeal, flour, baking powder, baking soda, and salt in a large bowl and stir to combine.

3. Place the milk, egg, honey, and oil in a small bowl and whisk to combine.

4. Pour liquid ingredients into cornmeal mixture and mix well. Scrape into the prepared pan, smoothing the top with a spatula. Bake until lightly browned and a tester comes out clean when inserted in the middle of the bread, 20 to 25 minutes.

Pasta Primavera (V) or Pasta Bolognese (F-Option)

This may look complicated, but once the vegetables are cleaned and trimmed, the wok makes quick work of the cooking. You can make the Bolognese sauce, if using, up to a day or two before and store, tightly covered in the refrigerator; bring it to room temperature and then heat as directed. The vegan sauce is whisked up and tossed with the vegetables and noodles at the last moment, and the measurements are easy to divide in half if you are planning to serve both the vegan and flex versions.

Makes 4 servings

■ **Vegan Sauce**

Makes 4 servings

4 tablespoons rice vinegar
4 tablespoons tamari or soy sauce
4 tablespoons vegetable broth or water
4 tablespoons coconut sugar or brown sugar
1 dried cayenne chile pepper, crumbled, or up to ½ teaspoon hot
    red pepper flakes
4 teaspoons cornstarch

■ *Bolognese Sauce*

Makes 4 servings

3 tablespoons extra-virgin olive oil or avocado oil
1 onion, chopped
4 garlic cloves, finely chopped
6 ounces ground lamb or chicken
6 tomatoes, coarsely chopped
½ cup grated Parmesan cheese
½ cup chopped fresh basil
1 dried cayenne chile pepper, crumbled or up to ½ teaspoon hot
 red pepper flakes

■ *Vegetables*

1 pound dry spaghetti or linguini
3 tablespoons extra-virgin olive oil or coconut oil
1 onion, cut in half, each half thickly sliced
1 leek, white and light green parts only, sliced
1 carrot, roughly chopped
1 red bell pepper, sliced
1 cup asparagus pieces or halved Brussels sprouts
1 cup sliced mushrooms
1 cup trimmed snow peas

1. Make the vegan sauce: Whisk the vinegar, tamari, broth, sugar, chile pepper, and cornstarch in a small bowl.

2. Make the Bolognese sauce: Heat the oil in a large skillet over medium-high heat. Add the onion and sauté about 4 minutes. Add the garlic and lamb and cook, stirring frequently and breaking up the meat with a wooden spoon, until the lamb is cooked through and there is no sign of pink, about 12 minutes. Add the tomatoes, cheese, basil, and chile; cook, stirring frequently, until the cheese has melted and the sauce thickens, about 6 minutes.

3. Cook the noodles: Bring a large pot of salted water to a boil over high heat. Add the noodles, cover, reduce the heat, and simmer until al dente, about 12 minutes. Drain the noodles, return them to the pot, and toss with 1 tablespoon of the oil; cover the pot and set aside.

4. Cook the vegetables: Heat the remaining 2 tablespoons of oil in a wok or large frying pan over high heat. Add the onion and leek and cook, stirring constantly, 2 minutes. Add the carrot and cook, stirring constantly, 2 minutes. Add the bell pepper, asparagus, and mushrooms and cook, stirring frequently, or until vegetables are crisp-tender, about 3 minutes.

5A. The Vegan Option: Stir the vegan sauce into the vegetables. Cook over medium-low heat, stirring constantly, until the sauce turns clear and thickens, about 2 minutes. Add the snow peas, reduce the heat to low, and add the noodles, tossing to mix with the vegetables until heated through, 1 or 2 minutes.

5B. The Flex Option: Stir the Bolognese sauce into the vegetables. Cook over medium-low heat, stirring constantly, until heated through, 1 to 2 minutes. Add the snow peas, reduce the heat to low, and add the noodles, tossing to mix with the vegetables and sauce. Stir until heated through, 1 or 2 minutes.

5C. For Both Options: Heat half of the Bolognese sauce in a large saucepan over medium-low heat. Add half of the cooked vegetables and half of the noodles and toss to combine. Cover and keep warm over low heat. Just before serving, add half the snow peas and heat through, about 30 seconds to 1 minute.

Stir half of the vegan sauce into the remaining vegetables in the wok. Cook, stirring constantly, until the sauce turns clear and thickens, 1 to 2 minutes. Add the remaining snow peas, reduce the heat to low, and add the remaining noodles, tossing to mix with the vegetables until heated through, about 30 seconds to 1 minute.

Soba Noodles with Pistachio Leeks (V) + Scallops (F-Option)

This dish is typically served warm or even chilled, but not usually hot, and so it works well as a flexible, meat-option dish because all the vegetables can be cooked and tossed with the noodles and set aside while the scallops are cooked. Scallops are best served immediately. To make all 4 servings with scallops, you will need 12 scallops, 4 tablespoons cornstarch, and 4 to 6 tablespoons oil; you may need to cook the scallops in 2 or 3 batches.

Makes 4 servings

8 ounces soba noodles
1 tablespoon toasted sesame oil
1 tablespoon tamari or soy sauce
1 garlic clove, minced
1 tablespoon freshly grated ginger
2 tablespoons extra-virgin olive oil or coconut oil
1 small onion, chopped
1 leek, white and green parts, thinly sliced on the diagonal
1 small red bell pepper, sliced
6 stemmed shiitake mushrooms, finely sliced
½ pound fresh spinach or baby bok choy, halved and sliced
  lengthwise
½ cup shelled pistachio nuts

■ Flex Version

Makes 1 serving

3 sea scallops
2 teaspoons cornstarch
1 tablespoon coconut oil

1. Bring a large saucepan or stockpot of salted water to a boil over high heat. Add the noodles and cook, stirring occasionally, until al dente, 3 to 4 minutes. Drain the noodles and rinse under cool water and drain well. Transfer the noodles to a large bowl and toss with the sesame oil, tamari, garlic, and ginger.

2. Heat the oil in a medium skillet over medium-high heat. Add the onion and leek and sauté 6 minutes. Add the bell pepper and mushrooms and cook, stirring frequently, until the vegetables are tender-crisp, about 5 minutes. Add spinach, cover the pan, reduce the heat to medium-low, and cook until the spinach is wilted, about 2 minutes.

3. Add the vegetables to the noodles, tossing to combine. Garnish each serving with 2 tablespoons nuts.

3A. The Flex Option: Pat the scallops dry and place on a shallow dish. Dust with the cornstarch, covering both sides. Heat the oil in a small skillet over medium-high heat. Using tongs, place the scallops in the hot oil and sear until crispy brown on underside, about 2 minutes. Flip and cook until the scallops are opaque and crispy brown on the second side, 1 to 2 minutes. Add the scallops to one serving of noodles, vegetables, and nuts.

Vegetable Risotto (V, GF) + Ham (F-Option)

Named after a town in Italy, Arborio rice is short-grained and white and has a high starch content, making it perfect for creamy risotto. Make this risotto seasonal: use fresh fennel in winter; add 1 cup fresh spring peas, wild mushrooms, or asparagus in spring; 1 cup chopped summer squash or fresh beans in summer; and 1 cup chopped bell peppers or pumpkin for a delicious fall dish.

If you don't have vegetable broth, add a chopped carrot, quartered onion, and 6 whole cloves to the water as it simmers on the stove.

Makes 4 servings

4 cups vegetable broth (see recipe introduction)
2 tablespoons extra-virgin olive oil or avocado oil
1 fennel bulb, thinly sliced
2 garlic cloves, finely chopped
2 tablespoons chopped fresh rosemary
1 cup Arborio rice
4 ounces soft goat cheese (chèvre), cut into pieces
4 tablespoons shaved Parmesan cheese, optional

Flex Version

Makes 1 serving

2 ounces smoked ham, chopped

1. Bring the broth to a boil in a large saucepan over medium-high heat. Cover, reduce the heat to low, and maintain at a simmer.

2. Heat the oil in a deep, heavy saucepan over medium-high heat. Add the fennel and cook, stirring often, 3 minutes. Stir in the garlic, rosemary, and rice, and cook, stirring frequently, until rice is glass-like, about 3 minutes.

3. Using a ladle, add ½ cup of hot broth to the rice mixture. Cook, stirring constantly, until the broth has been absorbed. Continue adding the broth, ½ cup at time, stirring and cooking until the rice has absorbed most or all of the broth and is tender but slightly al dente, about 20 minutes.

4. Add the goat cheese and cook, stirring constantly, until it has melted. Ladle the risotto into shallow bowls and garnish each with 1 tablespoon of Parmesan shavings if using.

4A. The Flex Option: Ladle the risotto into 3 bowls. Add the ham to the remaining risotto in the saucepan and stir to mix well. Ladle the flex portion into a bowl. Garnish each with 1 tablespoon of Parmesan shavings if using.

Whole Grain–Greens Stir-Fry (V, GF)

Whole and ancient grains play a major role in reducetarian recipes because they offer satisfying fiber and nutty flavor and contribute plant proteins. While each whole grain is unique, most require twice their volume of water or broth to cook, and they can take anywhere from 40 minutes for wild rice to upward of an hour for wheat berries or Khorasan wheat kernels (Kamut). Look for whole grains in whole food or health food stores and some major supermarkets. You can use whole grain brown barley, spelt, wheat berries, or wild rice in this recipe, but if you can find Khorasan wheat, try it because of its sweet and buttery flavor, high protein, and rich nutrient content.

Makes 4 to 6 servings

Ginger Sauce

Makes ⅓ cup

3 tablespoons tamari or soy sauce
2 tablespoons coconut nectar or liquid honey
1 tablespoon rice vinegar
2 teaspoons grated fresh ginger
2 teaspoons toasted sesame oil

Stir-Fry

2 tablespoons extra-virgin coconut oil
1 onion, chopped
1 leek, white and light green parts only, sliced
2 garlic cloves, finely chopped
¼ cup white wine
1 cup chopped rutabaga or parsnip
1 cup chopped broccoli
1 cup chopped kale or Swiss chard
½ red or green bell pepper, chopped
2 cups cooked whole grains (see recipe introduction)

1. Make the ginger sauce: Whisk the tamari, nectar, vinegar, ginger, and oil in a small bowl until combined. Set aside.

2. Make the stir-fry: Heat the oil in a large wok or Dutch oven over medium-high heat. Add the onion and leek and sauté 5 minutes. Add the garlic and cook, stirring frequently, 3 minutes.

3. Add the wine and bring to a simmer. Add the rutabaga and broccoli and cook, stirring frequently, 4 minutes. Add the kale and bell pepper and cook, stirring frequently, until the vegetables are tender-crisp, 3 to 4 minutes.

4. Stir in the grains and ginger sauce. Cook, stirring constantly, until the sauce thickens and the grains are heated through, about 1 minute.

SIDES AND SAUCES

- Braised Apples and Cabbage
- Fruit Salsa
- Gado Gado (Peanut Sauce)
- Roasted Vegetable Medley
- Tomato Sauce
- Winter Root Purée

Braised Apples and Cabbage (V, GF)

Red and purple vegetables are high in anthocyanins, nutrients that play a critical role in our health because they help the body in its defense against inflammation and cancer-causing free-radicals. Eat up.

Makes 4 to 6 servings

2 tablespoons extra-virgin coconut oil
2 small red onions, thinly sliced
2 tablespoons caraway seeds or cumin seeds
8 cups thinly sliced red cabbage
2 apples, sliced
½ cup apple juice or water
¼ cup cider vinegar
2 tablespoons coconut sugar or brown sugar
Sea salt and freshly ground black pepper to taste

1. Heat the oil in a large Dutch oven or heavy stockpot over medium-high heat. Add the onions and cook, stirring frequently, until soft, about 5 minutes. Add the caraway seeds, cabbage, and apples and stir or toss to combine.

2. Add the juice, vinegar, and sugar and bring to a boil. Cover, reduce the heat, and simmer, stirring frequently, until cabbage is tender, 25 to 35 minutes Season with salt and pepper.

Fruit Salsa (V, GF)

Pit, peel, and slice the peaches over the saucepan so that all their juices collect in the pan. Use any fresh summer berry: raspberries, strawberries, or blueberries or even pitted cherries in this piquant, sweet-sour relish. Serve it with Tofu Scramble (page 241), Green Rice Stir-Fry (page 274) or as a topping for Cheesy Apple Pancakes (page 235) or Mushroom Nut Burgers (page 275).

Makes 6 cups

8 large fresh peaches or nectarines, peeled and sliced

3 cups berries (see recipe introduction)

1 medium red onion, thinly sliced

1 jalapeño pepper, finely chopped

1 cup lightly packed brown sugar

1 cup apple cider vinegar

½ cup golden raisins

Two 2-inch cinnamon sticks, each cut into 3 pieces

3 tablespoons chopped fresh or candied ginger

1 teaspoon kosher or pickling salt

1. Combine the peaches, berries, onion, jalapeño, brown sugar, vinegar, raisins, cinnamon, ginger, and salt in a large saucepan. Bring to a boil over medium-high heat. Reduce the heat to low and simmer, stirring occasionally, until the sauce thickens, about 1 hour. Test the thickness by dropping a spoonful onto a plate. Draw a spoon through the center of the mixture. If no liquid seeps into the middle, the salsa is thick enough. Continue to simmer, testing every 10 minutes, until thick.

2. Ladle the salsa into clean canning jars, leaving 1-inch headspace. Wipe the rims clean and cover with the flat canning lid. Screw the ring on the jar just until comfortably tight. Let jars cool completely. Store in the refrigerator for up to 3 weeks or in the freezer for up to 3 months.

Gado Gado (Peanut Sauce) (V, GF)

With its origins in Indonesia, this sauce enhances the taste of grilled tofu or tempeh and is typically used to flavor thin strips of fish, chicken, or beef threaded onto skewers and roasted over hot coals. I love it tossed with steamed or roasted vegetables (see Roasted Vegetable Medley on page 266) or smeared over whole grain toast. If you make it and keep it in a covered jar in the refrigerator, you will find many ways to add it to dishes either before or after cooking.

For an easy lunch or dinner dish, toss up any/all of the following and drizzle Gado Gado sauce over: cooked potatoes, hard-boiled eggs, firm silken tofu, bok choy, steamed green beans or broccoli spears, quartered tomatoes, sliced radishes, cubed cucumber, avocado chunks, chopped sweet onion, spinach, or chopped kale. Peanuts and other nuts are often dusted with cornstarch or wheat flour, so check labels if you are gluten sensitive.

Makes 1½ cups

1 cup salted peanuts
3 garlic cloves, finely chopped
2 tablespoons extra-virgin coconut oil
1 small onion, chopped
½ cup vegetable broth
2 tablespoons rice vinegar
2 tablespoons tamari or soy sauce
2 tablespoons coconut nectar or liquid honey
1 tablespoon grated fresh ginger
1 or 2 fresh red chiles, optional

1. Place the peanuts and garlic in the bowl of a food processor and process until chopped very fine.

2. Heat the oil in a medium saucepan or skillet over medium-high heat. Add the onion and sauté until soft, 5 minutes.

3. Add the peanut mixture and broth. Bring to a boil and add the vinegar, tamari, coconut nectar, ginger, and chiles if using. Reduce the heat to low and simmer 5 minutes. Use immediately or transfer to a lidded container and store in the refrigerator for up to 5 days or freeze for up to 3 months.

Roasted Vegetable Medley (V, GF)

Root vegetables (potatoes, onions, beets, carrots, turnip, garlic, parsnips, rutabaga, sunchokes) and cruciferous vegetables (green cabbage, Brussels sprouts, broccoli, cauliflower) are delicious when roasted. The long, dry heat facilitates the change from starch or carbohydrates to sugar. Just a light coat of oil, a sprinkling of coarse salt, and some robust herbs are all that is needed to make a royal feast.

Makes 4 servings

3 to 4 cups 1- or 2-inch chunks of vegetables (see recipe
    introduction)
2 tablespoons melted extra-virgin coconut oil or olive oil
2 tablespoons chopped fresh rosemary, sage, and thyme blend or
    Green Herb Pesto (page 232)
1 tablespoon coarse salt

1. Preheat the oven to 400°F.

2. Toss the vegetables, oil, herbs, and salt in an 11 by 17-inch baking pan until combined. Roast, stirring once, until the vegetables are tender and golden brown, about 30 minutes.

Tomato Sauce (V, GF)

A good tomato sauce is so much more flavorful than anything in a can or jar. However, I must admit that except for late summer and early fall, when fresh heirloom tomatoes are pouring out of my garden and flooding farmers' markets, I do rely on tomatoes in glass jars (or BPA-free canned tomatoes) to make this sauce.

You can make a meal by simmering tempeh slices, tofu cubes, or boneless skinless chicken breasts in this sauce. Toss it with noodles and cheese or spread on pizza dough and dot with slices of baby mozzarella cheese for a fine Margherita pizza.

Makes about 3 cups

2 tablespoons extra-virgin olive oil or avocado oil
1 large onion, chopped
4 garlic cloves, finely chopped
6 to 10 large tomatoes, quartered, or 1 jar (28 ounces) diced
    tomatoes and juice
½ cup chopped fresh parsley
¼ cup chopped fresh basil
2 tablespoons chopped fresh rosemary
2 tablespoons chopped fresh thyme
1 tablespoon coarse sea salt

1. Heat the oil in a large heavy saucepan over medium-high heat. Add the onion and sauté 5 minutes. Add the garlic and cook, stirring frequently, until transparent and fragrant, about 2 minutes. Using a sharp paring knife and working over the pan, peel the skin away from each tomato quarter one at a time, discarding the skin. Coarsely chop the flesh, letting the pieces and juice run into the pan. Repeat with remaining quarters.

2. Bring the sauce to a boil, reduce the heat, and simmer until it has thickened slightly, 3 to 5 minutes. Stir in the parsley, basil, rosemary, thyme, and salt and simmer until blended, about 1 minute.

3. Use immediately or transfer to a lidded container and store in the refrigerator for up to 3 days or freeze for up to 3 months.

Winter Root Purée (V, GF)

Even those people that say they don't like parsnips enjoy this silky, sweet mash. You can make it chunky and fluffy or smooth and spreadable. You can spoon it alongside a main dish or plop it into a lettuce cup or spread it in a thin, round layer as a bed for a main dish. I love it so much I can be found spooning it right out of the pot!

Makes 2 to 4 servings

2 carrots, cut into 1-inch pieces

2 parsnips, cut into 1-inch pieces

1 cup 1-inch chunks rutabaga

2 tablespoons soft coconut oil or butter

1 tablespoon maple syrup or liquid honey, optional

1 teaspoon sea salt

1. Bring a large saucepan of salted water to a boil over high heat. Add the carrots, parsnips, and rutabaga and bring back to a boil. Partially cover, reduce the heat to medium-low, and simmer until the vegetables are soft, about 15 minutes.

2. Drain the vegetables and return them to the hot pot. Place the pot on hot burner with the heat turned off. Add the oil, maple syrup if using, and salt. Using a potato masher, mash the vegetables until they are the desired consistency. If you want a silky texture, use an immersion blender or process in batches in a food processor or blender.

MAINS AND CORE MEALS

- Autumn Vegetable Gratin
- Beans and Rice
- Chili-Veg Bowl or Turkey Chili
- Eggplant Buddha Bowl + Fish
- Curried Green Rice Stir-Fry + Shrimp
- Mushroom Nut Burgers or Loaf
- Pat's Pad Thai + Chicken

Autumn Vegetable Gratin (GF, V-Option)

Winter squash is a hardy vegetable that may be stored in a cool basement, garage, or cold cellar for months. In fact, this is one of the foods that sustained both Native Americans and newcomers to the New World through long, harsh winters. Choose from a variety of beautiful varieties of squash, such as ambercup, hokkaido, autumn cup, acorn, butternut,

hubbard, banana, buttercup, sweet potato, carnival, delicata, gold nug-
get, kabocha, sweet dumpling, and turban. Try them all and become a
squash connoisseur.

Makes 6 to 8 servings

1 cup shredded cheddar cheese, optional
¼ cup large-flake rolled oats
¼ cup chopped nuts (almond, walnut, pecan, or pistachio)
3 tablespoons chickpea or rice flour
1 tablespoon coconut sugar or brown sugar, optional
1 tablespoon dried rosemary or thyme
1 teaspoon coarse sea salt
1½ pounds winter squash, peeled, sliced, and seeded (see recipe
   introduction)
1 onion, sliced
3 small to medium potatoes, sliced
2 to 3 cups dairy or nut milk
½ cup grated Parmesan cheese, optional

1. Preheat the oven to 350°F. Oil a 2-quart baking dish.

2. Place the cheddar cheese if using, oats, nuts, flour, sugar if using,
rosemary, and salt in a small bowl; stir to combine. Set aside.

3. Layer one third of the squash, onion, and potatoes in the prepared baking dish. Sprinkle one third of the oat mixture over. Repeat the layers two more times, finishing with the oat mixture.

4. Pour enough of the milk over the vegetables to come two thirds
of the way up the sides of the baking dish. Using the back of a
wooden spoon, press down slightly to moisten all the ingredients.
Sprinkle Parmesan over the top if using. Bake until the vegetables
are tender and the top is bubby and golden brown, about 1 hour. If
the top browns before the vegetables are tender, cover with a lid or
foil. Remove from the oven and let stand covered for 15 minutes
before serving.

Beans and Rice (V, GF)

Almost every culture has an economical and nourishing traditional grain and bean dish. In Spain, the staple is known as arroz e feijão, the Haitians love their avas kon arroz, and the southern comfort food of Louisiana features red beans and homegrown rice. The beans are a perfect substitute for meat, but you can add a small amount of cooked chicken or fish to make this a flex dish.

The recipe calls for cooked rice and beans. If you are cooking dried beans, you need to allow a couple of hours and follow the recipe on page 244. Directions for cooking rice are included in step 2.

Makes 4 servings

2 cups cooked beans or 1 can (16 ounces, BPA-free) red, black or
   other beans
2 cups cooked brown rice (or 1 cup raw; see step 2)
3 tablespoons extra-virgin coconut oil
1 onion, chopped
¼ red cabbage, chopped
1 parsnip, chopped
1 carrot, chopped
3 garlic cloves, finely chopped
1 cup halved red grapes
2 tablespoons tamari or soy sauce
2 tablespoons balsamic vinegar
1 cup torn fresh spinach leaves

1. Cook the beans as described on page 244 or drain and rinse the canned beans and set aside.

2. To cook the rice: Bring 2 cups of salted water to a boil in a large saucepan over high heat. Add 1 cup rice, cover, reduce the heat, and simmer until the rice is tender, about 40 minutes. Fluff with a fork and set aside.

3. Heat the oil in a large saucepan over medium-high heat. Add the onion and sauté until soft, about 5 minutes. Add the cabbage, parsnip, carrot, garlic, and grapes and cook, stirring frequently, 5 minutes.

4. Add the tamari and vinegar and heat through. Reduce the heat to medium-low, stir in the spinach, cover, and cook until the leaves are wilted, about 1 minute. Add the beans, tossing to combine, and heat through.

5. Spoon the rice into individual bowls and top with the bean mixture.

Chili-Veg Bowl (V, GF) or Turkey Chili (F-Option)

As with many casseroles, the vegan version of this chili is better the next day. Don't skip the cumin and coriander because they are essential to the traditional chili flavor. You could add coarsely chopped tempeh for extra texture if you like. Kenearly and Aztec kidney beans are the varieties I use in this chili, but use whatever your market provides.

Makes 4 to 6 servings

1 cup mixed dried beans (see recipe introduction) or 1 can (16 ounces BPA-free) cooked kidney beans, rinsed and drained

3 tablespoons extra-virgin coconut oil

1 onion, chopped

½ red bell pepper, chopped

2 cups chopped mushrooms

3 garlic cloves, finely chopped

1 jalapeño pepper, finely chopped

1 jar (or BPA-free can) (28 ounces) diced or strained tomatoes and juices

¼ cup dark molasses

1 carrot, chopped

1 sweet potato, cut into 1-inch pieces

1 tablespoon sea salt

1 tablespoon ground cumin

2 teaspoons ground coriander

1 teaspoon chili powder

Ground Turkey (F-Option)

Makes 2 to 3 servings

1 tablespoon extra-virgin olive oil or coconut oil
½ pound ground turkey

1. If using dried beans allow several hours for soaking and cooking. Follow the cooking instructions on page 244.

2. Heat the oil in a soup pot over medium-high heat. Add the onion and sauté 5 minutes. Add the bell pepper and mushrooms and cook, stirring frequently, 5 minutes.

3. Stir in garlic and jalapeño pepper and cook, stirring frequently, 1 minute. Add the tomatoes and their juices, molasses, carrot, potato, salt, cumin, coriander, and chili powder. Bring to a boil, reduce the heat, and simmer, stirring occasionally, until the vegetables are tender, about 20 minutes.

4A. The Vegan Option: Stir in the cooked beans and heat through.

4B. The Flex Option: While the sauce is cooking, heat the oil in a large skillet over medium-high heat. Add the turkey, reduce the heat to medium, and cook, breaking up the meat and stirring frequently with a wooden spoon, until meat has browned with no sign of pink, 10 to 12 minutes. Ladle one half of the vegetable chili into the cooked turkey and mix well.

Eggplant Buddha Bowl (V, GF) + Fish (F-Option)

Although this is not a bitingly hot spicy dish, the coconut and garam masala along with the cinnamon, cayenne, and ginger warm it. When the flavors have a chance to mellow overnight, the result is richly layered and complex.

Makes 4 to 6 servings

¼ cup extra-virgin coconut oil

2 onions, chopped

1 small eggplant, cut into 1-inch cubes

3 garlic cloves, finely chopped

1 medium zucchini, chopped

½ red bell pepper, chopped

3 or 4 chopped fresh tomatoes

Two 2-inch cinnamon sticks

1 or 2 cayenne peppers, finely chopped

1 tablespoon Garam Masala Spice Blend (page 231)

1 teaspoon sea salt

½ teaspoon freshly ground black pepper

2 tablespoons grated fresh ginger

1 can (15 ounces) coconut milk

10 small potatoes, halved

½ cup water

Fish (F-Option)

Makes 2 servings

1 whitefish fillet (6 to 8 ounces)

1. Heat the oil in a large saucepan or skillet over medium-high heat. Add the onions and eggplant and sauté until soft, 5 minutes. Add the garlic, zucchini, and bell pepper and cook, stirring frequently, until the vegetables are tender-crisp, about 6 minutes.

2. Stir in the tomatoes, cinnamon, cayenne peppers, spice blend, salt, black pepper, ginger, and coconut milk and bring to a boil over high heat.

3. Add the potatoes and the water if the sauce is too dry. Cover, reduce the heat to medium-low, and cook until the potatoes are tender, about 12 minutes.

3A. The Flex Option: Spoon 3 cups of the coconut-potato mixture into a separate pan. Add the fish and some extra water if the sauce is too dry. Cover, reduce the heat to medium-low, and simmer until the fish is cooked (it turns opaque and flakes easily with a fork), 6 to 10 minutes.

Curried Green Rice Stir-Fry (V, GF) + Shrimp (F-Option)

Like all grains, rice that is the least processed will provide the most nutrients. I love the nutty flavor of red, mahogany, black, and brown short-grain rice and I keep many of them in my pantry all the time. Wild black rice may be added to any rice blend. Because it includes the natural bran and germ, whole grain rice takes a while to cook and always retains a chewy texture.

Makes 4 to 6 servings

3 tablespoons extra-virgin coconut oil
1 onion, chopped
1 carrot, chopped
½ red bell pepper, chopped
6 mushrooms, chopped
1 small zucchini, chopped
1 cup mixed red, brown, and wild rice
1 tablespoon Red Curry Paste (page 233)
2 cups vegetable broth or water
1 head broccoli, thinly sliced
1 cup Brussels sprouts, thinly sliced
1 cup Gado Gado sauce (page 265), optional

Shrimp (F-Option)

Serves 1

4 jumbo shrimp, peeled and deveined

1. Heat the oil in a large skillet or casserole pan over medium-high heat. Add the onion and sauté 4 minutes. Add the carrot and bell pepper and cook, stirring frequently, 2 minutes. Add the mushrooms and zucchini and cook, stirring frequently, 3 minutes.

2. Add the rice and curry paste and cook, stirring constantly, 1 minute. Add the broth and bring to a boil, stirring frequently. Cover, reduce the heat, and simmer 30 minutes.

3. Spread the broccoli and Brussels sprouts evenly over the top of the rice mixture. Cover and simmer until the rice is tender and the vegetables are tender-crisp, about 10 minutes. Serve with Gado Gado sauce if desired.

3A. The Flex Option: Bring 3 cups of water to a boil in a medium saucepan. Add the shrimp, reduce the heat, and simmer gently until the shrimp turn bright pink, about 3 minutes. Remove from the pan using tongs and add to one serving of the stir-fry.

Mushroom Nut Burgers or Loaf (V-Option, GF)

The eggs act as a binder for the ingredients. To make this a vegan dish, use 2 tablespoons chia seeds soaked in ¼ cup water or an egg alternative instead. This is one of my finest vegetarian burger/meat loaf recipes and I hope you agree.

Makes 4 burgers or one 9 by 5-inch loaf

3 tablespoons extra-virgin coconut or olive oil

1 onion, chopped

3 garlic cloves, finely chopped

1 red bell pepper, chopped

1 zucchini, chopped

2 cups chopped mushrooms

1 cup chopped cashew nuts

1 cup quinoa flakes or large-flaked rolled oats

¼ cup Tomato Sauce (page 266) or prepared

2 eggs, lightly beaten (see recipe introduction)

1 tablespoon chopped fresh thyme

1 teaspoon sea salt

1. Heat the oil in a medium saucepan or skillet over medium-high heat. Add the onion and sauté 5 minutes. Add the garlic, bell pepper, zucchini, and mushrooms and cook, stirring frequently, until vegetables are soft, about 5 minutes. Set aside to cool slightly.

2. Preheat the oven to 350°F. Line a baking sheet with parchment paper (for burgers) or oil a 9 by 5-inch loaf pan.

3. Place the nuts, quinoa, tomato sauce, eggs, thyme, and salt in a large bowl, stirring to combine. Add the vegetable mixture and mix well.

4A. The Burger Option: Place 1 cup of the mixture onto the prepared baking sheet and pat into a 1-inch-thick patty. Repeat with the remaining burger mixture. Bake until browned on the outside and cooked through, about 45 minutes. Let stand for 5 minutes before removing from the sheet.

4B. The Loaf Option: Transfer the burger mixture to the prepared loaf pan, smoothing the top with a spatula. Bake until browned on outside and cooked through, about 1 hour. Let stand for 5 minutes before removing from the pan and slicing.

Pat's Pad Thai (V, GF) + Chicken (F-Option)

Give this some heat by adding crushed dried cayenne pepper or a finely chopped jalapeño pepper. It's a pretty versatile dish—you can omit the coconut milk, for example—and it's very easy to make because the noodles are ready by the time the rest of the ingredients are cooked in the wok.

Makes 6 servings

1 package (7 ounces) rice stick noodles

Vegan

3 tablespoons extra-virgin coconut oil or olive oil

1 yellow onion, chopped

1 red bell pepper, chopped

4 green onions, quartered lengthwise and cut into 1-inch lengths

2 cups sliced bok choy (white stems and green tops)

1 tablespoon toasted sesame oil

4 garlic cloves, finely chopped

1 round or 1-inch cube candied ginger, finely chopped

1 cup coconut milk

½ cup chili sauce

¼ cup freshly squeezed lime juice

4 ounces medium tofu, cubed

2 cups fresh bean sprouts, optional

1 cup salted pistachio nuts or peanuts

Chicken (F-Option)

Makes 2 servings

1 boneless, skinless chicken breast, cut into ½-inch strips

2 cups chicken broth or water

1. Place the noodles in a large bowl and pour boiling water over to cover. Set aside until plump and softened but not soggy, about 5 minutes. Drain and set aside in a large bowl.

2. Heat 2 tablespoons of coconut oil in a large wok or skillet over medium-high heat. Add the yellow onion and sauté 4 minutes. Add the bell pepper, green onions, and bok choy and cook, stirring frequently, until the vegetables are tender-crisp, about 4 minutes. Using a slotted spoon, transfer the vegetables to the bowl with the noodles; toss to combine.

3. Heat the remaining 1 tablespoon coconut oil and the sesame oil in the wok. Add the garlic and ginger and cook, stirring constantly, 1 minute. Add the coconut milk, chili sauce, and lime juice and bring to a boil. Reduce the heat and simmer until the sauce thickens slightly, 2 to 3 minutes.

4A. The Vegan Option: Add tofu and noodles mixture to the wok, toss to combine, and heat through. Using tongs, plate the pad thai and garnish with the bean sprouts if using and nuts.

4B. The Flex Option: While the sauce is cooking, bring the broth or water to a boil in a medium saucepan over high heat. Add the chicken, reduce the heat, and simmer the chicken until cooked through, about 6 minutes. Remove the chicken from the cooking liquid and divide evenly between 2 servings of pad thai. Garnish with the bean sprouts if using and nuts.

SWEETS

- Apple Crisp
- Baked Chocolate Rice Pudding
- Blender Carrot Cake
- Cream Cheese Frosting
- Blueberries and Cashew Cream
- Chocolate-Coconut Chunk Cookies

Apple Crisp (V, GF)

Of course, you can eliminate the sugar by substituting liquid honey, brown rice syrup, coconut nectar, or pure maple syrup. They all have a distinctly different flavor, so each time you make this, try a different sugar alternative and get to know how each tastes in desserts.

Makes 4 to 6 servings

Crisp Topping
2 cups finely chopped almonds or pecans

2 cups large-flake rolled oats or quinoa flakes

½ cup packed coconut sugar or brown sugar

2 tablespoons chickpea or rice flour

1 teaspoon ground cinnamon

½ teaspoon sea salt

½ cup softened extra-virgin coconut oil or butter

Apple Filling

  3 tablespoons packed coconut sugar or brown sugar

  2 tablespoons chickpea or rice flour

  6 to 8 apples, quartered

  3 tablespoons extra-virgin coconut oil or butter, cut into pieces

1. Preheat the oven to 350°F. Lightly oil a 3-quart baking dish.

2. Make the topping: Combine the almonds, oats, sugar, flour, cinnamon, and salt in a medium bowl. Using a pastry blender or your hands, work the coconut oil into the flour mixture until the pieces are about the size of peas.

3. Make the filling: Combine the sugar and flour in a large bowl. Add the quartered apples to the sugar mixture and toss to mix well. Transfer the apples to the prepared dish and dot with the oil.

4. Crumble the crisp topping evenly over the fruit. Bake until the fruit is soft and the topping is bubbly and lightly browned, about 40 minutes.

Baked Chocolate Rice Pudding (V-Option, GF)

You can use rice milk or almond milk or half-and-half dairy milk in this recipe. Dark chocolate (70 to 80 percent cacao) has antioxidant properties, so it is preferred over milk chocolate but it is bitter and that is why coconut sugar is included in the recipe. Serve warm for dessert. Cover tightly and refrigerate leftover pudding and serve with fresh fruit for breakfast or as a midday snack.

Makes 8 to 10 servings

  2 large eggs or egg substitute

  1 teaspoon vanilla extract

  1 teaspoon ground cinnamon

  ½ teaspoon sea salt

  2 cups nut milk (see recipe introduction)

  4 ounces semisweet or bittersweet dark chocolate, chopped

  ¾ cup coconut sugar or granulated sugar

  1½ cups cooked rice

1. Preheat the oven to 350°F. You will need a 1½-quart ungreased baking dish or Dutch oven and a deep baking pan that is large enough for the baking dish to sit within.

2. Beat eggs lightly in a large bowl. Whisk in the vanilla, cinnamon, and salt, and set aside.

3. Bring the milk to a simmer in a medium saucepan over medium heat. Add the chocolate, reduce the heat to medium-low, and cook, whisking constantly, until the chocolate has melted, about 3 minutes. Remove from the heat and add the sugar, stirring until it has melted. Bring a kettle of water to boil.

4. Stir the rice into the egg mixture. Add the chocolate mixture to the rice and egg mixture in a slow, thin stream, stopping frequently to mix well at first. When the chocolate and rice mixtures have been combined, scrape into the baking dish. Set the baking dish inside the baking pan and pour boiling water into the pan until it reaches about three quarters of the way up the outside of the baking dish. Bake until a knife inserted into the center comes out clean, 50 to 60 minutes.

Blender Carrot Cake (GF-Option)

Although moist and tender, this version isn't a traditional carrot cake because you won't see bits of carrot throughout. You can add ½ cup of coarsely chopped walnuts to the batter when you add the pineapple in step 3.
If you don't have a high-performance blender, use a food processor to blend the liquid ingredients, then simply stir them into the dry ingredients in the bowl.

   Makes one 9-inch cake

2 cups all-purpose flour or gluten-free flour blend

1 teaspoon baking powder

1 teaspoon ground cinnamon

1 teaspoon sea salt

½ teaspoon baking soda

¼ teaspoon ground nutmeg

3 carrots, cut into chunks

1 can (8 ounces) crushed pineapple and juices

2 large eggs

⅓ cup soft extra-virgin coconut oil

1 cup granulated sugar

Cream Cheese Frosting (below) or Cashew Cream (page 282), optional

1. Preheat the oven to 375°F. Lightly oil a 9 by 9-inch baking pan.

2. Whisk the flour, baking powder, cinnamon, salt, baking soda, and nutmeg in a medium bowl.

3. Place carrots in a blender container and pulse until chopped, about 30 seconds. Add the pineapple and juices, eggs, oil, and sugar, and pulse until well mixed, about 1 minute. Add the flour mixture and pulse just until mixed, about 15 seconds.

4. Scrape the batter into the prepared pan. Bake 30 minutes. Reduce the heat to 350°F and bake until a cake tester inserted into the center comes out clean, about 15 minutes. Let the cake cool in the pan on a wire cooling rack. Remove to a cake plate and serve warm or let cool completely and ice the top with Cream Cheese Frosting or Cashew Cream if desired.

Cream Cheese Frosting (GF)

½ cup (4 ounces) cream cheese, softened

2 tablespoons soft extra-virgin coconut oil

Juice and grated rind of half a lemon

1½ to 2 cups confectioners' sugar

1. Beat the cheese and oil in a medium bowl using a wooden spoon. Beat in the lemon juice and lemon rind.

2. Beat in the sugar, ½ cup at a time, until the mixture is smooth and spreadable.

Blueberries and Cashew Cream (V, GF, R)

This cream is a staple vegan spread or topping. Unsweetened, it may be used as a substitute for cream cheese, whipped cream, and sour cream in most recipes. I've added some coconut sugar to it, so it is darker than the unsweetened version. It's easy to make but don't try to skip the soaking step.

Makes 3 cups cashew cream, 4 to 6 servings

2 cups raw cashews
2 cups boiling water
¼ to ½ cup coconut sugar, optional
½ cup fresh cool water
2 cups blueberries or other seasonal berries

1. Place the cashews in a large bowl and pour the boiling water over top. Cover with a kitchen towel and set aside for 6 to 8 hours or overnight.

2. Drain and transfer the nuts to a blender container. Add the sugar if using and ½ cup cool water. Blend on high until smooth and the consistency of sour cream, about 4 minutes. Add more water, 1 tablespoon at a time, and pulse 30 seconds if the mixture is too stiff.

3. Divide the berries among 4 or 6 bowls and spoon a dollop of cashew cream over top. Cover the leftover cream tightly and keep in the refrigerator for up to 1 week.

Chocolate-Coconut Chunk Cookies (GF-Option)

I like to blend the ingredients by hand but if you wish to use a stand mixer, do not add the chocolate or coconut to the flour mixture in step 2. Beat the coconut oil and egg mixture as directed in step 3 and then gradually add the flour mixture, beating until combined. Remove the bowl from the mixer and fold the chocolate and coconut into the dough using a spatula and continue with steps 5 and 6.

Makes 1 dozen cookies

2½ cups all-purpose or gluten-free blend flour
1½ teaspoons baking soda
1 teaspoon sea salt
½ teaspoon baking powder
3 cups semisweet chocolate chunks
1¼ cups coconut chunks or coarsely-chopped dried cherries
1 cup soft extra-virgin coconut oil or butter
¾ cup granulated sugar
½ cup packed coconut sugar or brown sugar
2 large eggs
2 teaspoons pure vanilla extract

1. Arrange 2 oven racks in the center of the oven. Preheat the oven to 350°F. Lightly oil two baking sheets or line with parchment paper.

2. Whisk the flour, baking soda, salt, and baking powder in a medium bowl until combined. Stir in the chocolate and coconut.

3. Beat the oil and granulated sugar in a large bowl until combined. Beat in the brown sugar and the eggs, one at a time, until the mixture is fluffy and well combined. Beat in the vanilla.

4. Sprinkle 1 cup of the flour mixture over the oil-sugar mixture and stir until combined. Repeat until all of the flour mixture is blended into the oil-sugar mixture.

5. Scoop about ¼ cup of the dough and drop onto the prepared baking sheets, spacing the cookies about 1½ inches apart.

6. Using two racks, bake 7 minutes. Rotate the baking sheets front to back and top to bottom and continue to bake until the cookies are golden around the edges, 8 to 10 minutes. Set aside on a wire cooling rack for a couple of minutes before transferring the cookies directly to the rack to cool completely. Store in an airtight container for up to 5 days at room temperature.

NOTES

INTRODUCTION

1. Orlich, M. J., Singh, P. N., Sabate, J., et al. (2013). Vegetarian Dietary Patterns and Mortality in Adventist Health Study 2. *JAMA Internal Medicine, 173*, 1230–1238.
2. Dur, J. (2015, March 11). Holy Cow! Meat Eaters Consume 7,000 Animals in Lifetime. *USA Today*. Retrieved from usatoday.com/story/news/nation-now/2015/03/11/meat-eaters-animals-lifetime/70136010.
3. Hoekstra, A. Y. (2012). The Hidden Water Resource Use behind Meat and Dairy. *Animal Frontiers, 2*(2), 3–8.
4. Tilman, D., & Clark, M. (2014). Global Diets Link Environmental Sustainability and Human Health. *Nature, 515*, 518–522.

THE BIZARRE FORCES THAT DRIVE PEOPLE TO EAT TOO MUCH MEAT

1. USDA. (2003). Profiling Food Consumption in America. In *U.S. Department of Agriculture Fact Book 2001–2002*. Washington, DC: U.S. Government Printing Office. Retrieved from usda.gov/factbook/index.html.
2. Rivera-Ferre, Marta. (2009). Supply vs. Demand of Agri-industrial Meat and Fish Products: A Chicken and Egg Paradigm. *Int. Jrnl. of Soc. of Agr. & Food, 16*(2), 90–105.

THE ELEMENT OF SURPRISE

1. Villarica, H. (2012, April 9). The Chocolate-and-Radish Experiment That Birthed the Modern Conception of Willpower. *The Atlantic*. Retrieved from theatlantic.com/health/archive/2012/04/the-chocolate-and-radish-experiment-that-birthed-the-modern-conception-of-willpower/255544.
2. Schultz, W. (2000). Multiple Reward Signals in the Brain. *Nature Reviews. Neuroscience, 1*(3), 199–207.
3. Subramanian, C. (2013, September 3). Google Study Gets Employees to Stop Eating So Many M&Ms. *Time*. Retrieved from newsfeed.time.com/2013/09/03/google-study-gets-employees-to-stop-eating-so-many-mms.

A LITTLE LESS LONELY IN MY CORNER OF THE WORLD

1. Wood, M. (2014, December 31). Recycling Electronic Waste Responsibly: Excuses Dwindle. *The New York Times*. Retrieved from nytimes.com/2015/01/01/technology/personaltech/recycling-electronic-waste-responsibly-excuses-dwindle.html.

CANNIBALISM IS NATURAL TOO

1. Stoneking, M. (2003). Widespread Prehistoric Human Cannibalism: Easier to Swallow? *Trends in Ecology and Evolution, 18*, 489–490.

A NUDGE IN THE RIGHT DIRECTION

1. Johnson, E. J., & Goldstein, D. (2003). Do Defaults Save Lives? *Science, 302*(5649), 1338–1339.
2. Wansink, B., Painter, J. E., & North, J. (2005). Bottomless Bowls: Why Visual Cues of Portion Size May Influence Intake. *Obesity Research, 13*(1) 93–100. Retrieved from foodpsychology.cornell.edu/research/bottomless -bowls-why-visual-cues-portion-size-may-influence-intake.
3. Levin, I. P., & Gaeth, G. (1998). How Consumers Are Affected by the Framing of Attribute Information before and after Consuming the Product. *Journal of Consumer Research, 15*, 374–378. Retrieved from jcr.oxfordjournals.org/content/15/3/374.

WHY WE CRAVE MEAT IN THE FIRST PLACE

1. Haddad, E. H., & Tanzman, J. S. (2003). What Do Vegetarians in the United States Eat? *American Journal of Clinical Nutrition, 78*(3), 626S–632S.
2. Fraser, G. E., & Shavlik D. J. (2001). Ten Years of Life. *JAMA Internal Medicine, 161*, 1645–1652.

EFFECTIVE REDUCETARIANISM

1. Norwood, F. B., & Lusk, J. (2011). *Compassion, by the Pound: The Economics of Farm Animal Welfare.* New York: Oxford University Press.

HOW MUCH MEAT ARE WE DESIGNED TO EAT?

1. Gibbons, A. (2013, February). The Evolution of Diet. *National Geographic.* Retrieved from nationalgeographic.com/foodfeatures/evolution-of-diet.

THE CHALLENGE OF FEEDING LESS MEAT TO DOGS AND CATS

1. Axelsson, E. (2013, March 21). The Genomic Signature of Dog Domestication Reveals Adaptation to a Starch-Rich Diet. *Nature, 495*(7441): 360–364.
2. Brown, W. Y., Vanselow, B. A., Redman, A. J., & Pluske, J. R. (2009, November). An Experimental Meat-Free Diet Maintained Haematological Characteristics in Sprint-Racing Sled Dogs. *British Journal of Nutrition, 102*(9), 1318–1323.

HOW TO LIVE LONG AND DIE WELL

1. Disclaimer: I am the book's co-author.
2. Ornish, D., Lin J., Chan, J. M., Epel, E., et al. (2013). Effect of Comprehensive Lifestyle Changes on Telomerase Activity and Telomere Length in Men with Biopsy-Proven Low-Risk Prostate Cancer: 5-Year Follow-Up of a Descriptive Pilot Study. *Lancet Oncology, 14*(11), 1112–1120.

SEEKING THE OPTIMAL DIET TO MAXIMIZE DISEASE REVERSAL AND LONGEVITY

1. Levine, M., Suarez, J., Brandhorst, S., et al. (2014). Low Protein Intake Is Associated with a Major Reduction in IGF-1, Cancer, and Overall Mortality in the 65 and Younger but Not Older Population. *Cell Metabolism, 19*(3), 407–417.
2. Fuhrman, J., Sarter, B., Glaster, B., & Acocella, S. (2010). Changing perceptions of hunger on a high nutrient density diet. *Nutritional Journal, 9,* 51.

ANTIBIOTIC RESISTANCE AT THE MEAT COUNTER

1. U.S. Department of Health and Human Services. (2013, April). *Antibiotic Resistance Threats in the United States 2013.* Atlanta: Centers for Disease Control and Prevention Office of Infectious Disease.
2. Rogers, L. (2016, January 29). Will Yum! Brands Commit to Better Antibiotic Stewardship Policies? *The Huffington Post.* Retrieved from huffingtonpost.com/laura-rogers/will-yum-brands-commit-to_b_9095108.html.

LESS MEAT TAKES A BITE OUT OF GLOBAL HUNGER

1. Cassidy, E., West, P., Gerber, J., & Foley, J. (2013, September). Redefining Agricultural Yields: From Tonnes to People Nourished Per Hectare. *Environmental Research Letters, 8*(3), IOPScience.
2. Smil, V. (2013). *Should We Eat Meat: Evolution and Consequences of Modern Carnivory.* Chichester, UK: Wiley-Blackwell.

AN UNCERTAIN PHOSPHORUS FUTURE

1. Metson, G. S., Bennett, E. M., & Elser, J. J. (2012). The Role of Diet in Phosphorus Demand. *Environmental Research Letters, 7*(4), 044043.
2. Smith, V. H., & Schindler, D. W. (2009). Eutrophication Science: Where Do We Go from Here? *Trends in Ecology & Evolution, 24,* 201–207.

THE NITROGEN STORY

1. Sutton, M. A., Bleeker, A., Howard, C. M., et al. (2013). Our Nutrient World: The Challenge to Produce More Food and Energy with Less

Pollution. *Global Overview of Nutrient Management. Centre of Ecology and Hydrology.* Edinburgh: On behalf of the Global Partnership on Nutrient Management and the International Nitrogen Initiative.

2. Westhoek, H., Lesschen, J. P., Rood, T., et al. (2014). Food Choices, Health and Environment: Effects of Cutting Europe's Meat and Dairy Intake. *Global Environmental Change, 26,* 196–205.

FEEDING THE WORLD AND MAKING ROOM FOR ALL SPECIES

1. Cassidy, E. S. (2013). Redefining Agricultural Yields: From Tonnes to People Nourished per Hectare. *Environmental Research Letters, 8*(3), 034015.
2. Eshel, G. (2014). Land, Irrigation Water, Greenhouse Gas, and Reactive Nitrogen Burdens of Meat, Eggs, and Dairy Production in the United States. *Proceedings of the National Academy of Sciences, 111*(33) 11996–12001.
3. Foley, J. A. (2011). Solutions for a Cultivated Planet. *Nature, 478*(7369) 337–342.

THE FOOD DESERT PHENOMENON

1. Cummins, S., & Macintyre, S. (2002). A Systematic Study of an Urban Foodscape: The Price and Availability of Food in Greater Glasgow. *Urban Studies, 39,* 2115–2130.

THE GLOBAL MAP OF WHO EATS TOO MUCH MEAT

1. Chappell, B. (2011, November 3). Along with Humans, Who Else Is in the 7 Billion Club? National Public Radio. Retrieved from npr.org/sections/thetwo-way/2011/11/03/141946751/along-with-humans-who-else-is-in-the-7-billion-club.
2. Stotesbury, N., & Dorling, D. (2015, October 21). Understanding Income Inequality and Its Implications: Why Better Statistics Are Needed. *Statistics Views.* Retrieved from http://www.statisticsviews.com/details/feature/8493411/Understanding-IncomeInequality-and-its-Implications-Why-Better-Statistics-Are-N.html.

ACKNOWLEDGMENTS

This book would not have been possible without the support and encouragement of (literally) hundreds of talented and gifted people. At the top of that list is my amazing and tireless literary agent, Linda Konner, who was willing to put in the time and effort required to work with a first-time author like myself. Words cannot express my gratitude to Sara Carder for her insightful advice on how best to polish this manuscript, to Brianna Yamashita and Keely Platte for their commitment to marketing and publicizing the book, to Joanna Ng for her thoughtful attention to detail and editorial assistance, to Nellys Liang for designing the stunning book cover, and to Pat Crocker for pouring her heart and soul into the fabulous recipes.

An enormous thank you goes out to Arthur E. Benjamin, Fabiola Beracasa, and Ashley Berrysmith for their invaluable mentorship and extraordinary vision. Thank you to Nancy Degnan, Jill Shapiro, Autumn Payne, Geoff Hempill, Joshua Drew, Jennifer Betancourt, Leah DeSole, Lisa French, Shahid Naeem, and Frank Wolf for helping me steer my ship in life. Further thanks go to Melissa Beveridge, Meredith Bennett-Smith, Leyla Acaroglu, Christine Hirt, Daniel Schwartz, Allegra DePasquale, Nina LoSchiavo, Carlyn Cowen, Seisei Tatebe-Goddu, Meira Harris, Cheyn Shah, Danika Lam, Emma Eytan, Sharon Wu, Richard Lee, Matthew Ashton, Cameron Shorb, Daisy Freund, Jenny Edwards, Georgie Mallet, Tyler Puckett, Krystal Caldwell, Bobbie Macdonald, Greg Boese, Peter Hurford, Sofia Davis-Fogel, Michelle Cone, Liv Boeree, Dalton Sweet, Anton Vallo, Max Elder, Rachel Atcheson, Alan Darer, Kyle Fujisawa, Mary Williams, Marcin Kowrygo, Jake Levin, Scott Weathers, Margaret Weinberg, Lauren Wolahan, Michael Trollan, Sylvia Wood, Derek Coons, Alice Cichon, Ailanit Davydova, Olaf Woldan, Jorge Lugo, and Sarah Brodie who volunteered their time and expertise to advance the Reducetarian movement.

This book really belongs to the countless essay contributors who spent a great deal of energy educating readers about the importance of eating fewer animal products. Thank you to my co-founder Tyler

Alterman, for his wacky suits and even wackier ideas. Thank you to my insane best friends—Michael Young, Dan Feldman, Isabella Cardona, David Di Lillo, Joe Eastman, Danielle Medina, Vincent Romano, Crichton Atkinson, Lauren Deaderick, Michelle Yakobson, Mark Barahman, David Craig, Michael Stivers, Arthur Kapetanakis, and Katina Boutis for their unwavering support. Thank you to my surrogate families—Sharon and Michael, Kim, Big Jeff, Little Jeff, and Chris, and Annie, Mark, Wesley, and Brittany—for their generosity and warmth.

Thank you to my loving mom and dad who have always been there for me and believed in me; to my sister, Jennifer, for challenging me at the dinner table; to Grandma Rose for teaching me to buy grapes only when they are on sale; and to Tobey for her companionship and for her loyalty.

And finally, a special thank you to Isabel, who reminds me there is always something to see if you know where to look, and inspires me to be a better person. I would never have made it this far without you by my side.

INDEX